MAXIMUM
IMMUNITY

MAXIMUM IMMUNITY

by

Michael A. Weiner, Ph.D.

with

Kathleen Goss, M.A.

616,079

4/86

1986

HOUGHTON MIFFLIN COMPANY

Boston

Library of Congress Cataloging in Publication Data

Weiner, Michael A.
Maximum immunity.

Bibliography: p.
Includes index.
1. Immunity—Nutritional aspects. 2. Immunologic
diseases—Popular works. 3. Immunology—Popular works.
I. Title.
QR185.2.W45   1985   616.07′9   85-18033
ISBN 0-395-37910-5

Printed in the United States of America

P   10   9   8   7   6   5   4   3   2   1

For Rebecca, Russell, and Janet, my immunity

Acknowledgments

Many colleagues helped me to understand the difficult field of immunology. I owe my gratitude to them and especially to Robert F. Cathcart III, M.D., for his inspired conversations, which brought me back in spirit to my first days in scientific discovery. All of the difficult facts would not have made a book without the masterful advice and perseverance of my editor, Mrs. Ruth Hapgood, who so artfully tended the volcano of information and controlled the flow of lava.

Contents

PART I

IMMUNITY

o 1 o

The Immunity Connection

IMMUNITY — the word itself is magic. Our immune system is the body's legacy from millions of years of evolution. It is a multipart, many-tiered, incredibly sophisticated system by which our bodies are able to naturally resist disease and infection — to fight off the invading bacteria, viruses, and other organisms that surround us constantly in our potentially hostile environment.

Maximum Immunity will show you how to use proper diet, vitamins, exercise, and plain common sense to enhance your body's natural immune system and make it as strong as it possibly can be. That will allow your own body and its defense systems to ward off and fight off simple illnesses such as the common cold and the flu. We will also show you how to build up your resistance to complex illnesses such as rheumatoid arthritis and AIDS.

But we are not talking about throwing away all of medical history. *Maximum Immunity* is about using all the natural nutritional devices that you can put your hands on simply to enhance and strengthen your body's own immune system and to show how you can use these in conjunction with the developments of modern science.

The problem with modern-day medicine — a problem acknowledged by most medical educators and thinkers themselves — is that it is a reactive medicine. Instead of focusing on the *prevention* of illness, modern medicine, and all its arsenal of pharmaceutical weapons, focuses on the disease *after* it invades the body and goes into battle with the immune system.

The age of antibiotics is fast coming to a close. Because of their great numbers, viruses and bacteria have quickly evolved resistant strains for almost every major manmade pharmaceutical. Positive preventive health is becoming more and more important.

How many people go to a doctor when they feel fine? Not many; you usually go to the doctor after you have become ill. And by then, it is generally too late to use your natural defenses alone to fight the disease because the invading bacterium or virus has already attacked you and is already locked in battle with your immune system. You can still benefit from adding nutritional "strengtheners" — vitamins, minerals, and amino acids — to your diet to help your immune system fight off the attack, but you may want the additional power of drugs at that late date, once the disease has already taken hold.

Maximum Immunity will show you how to use the most powerful weapons you have to strengthen your body's own resistance to illness. These are your mind, the food you eat, the exercise you get, and the rest you take — it really is almost that simple. Every major and minor disease eventually becomes a disease of the immune system, because the immune system incorporates the body's total response to illness — from early warning, to full-scale battle, to a state of siege. The result of human evolution is that our bodies have become finely tuned instruments that have the capability of fighting against almost every kind of invading organism or every internal disturbance. But once an invading microbe has taken hold, latched onto your body, and started to attack you within, you can not just add a couple of vitamins as supplements and expect your body to be able to repel that invading particle. At that point, large doses of specific immune-enhancing nutrients and a modified diet are essential. If that fails, drug therapy may be necessary; but even here, a solid immune-enhancing program should speed recovery.

But *Maximum Immunity* is about going beyond drugs. In Chapters 2 and 3, you will see in detail what your immune system consists of and how it works. Remember that a finely tuned immune system has to be provided with the proper vitamins, minerals, and other nutrients to operate at peak efficiency. And the irony of it all is that those of us who live in the most "developed" countries often have the most unbalanced diets. The manufacturing processes that provide us with convenience foods, that allow our food chains to be artificially manipulated, remove some of the essential elements of a balanced diet needed by our immune system. So in this, the most affluent nation in the world, more and more people have diets deficient in essential nutritional substances — substances whose importance to the immune system can be overwhelming. Modern urban man is overweight and malnourished, overstressed and unfit.

In the early part of the twentieth century, the prevailing wisdom called for treating the invading microbe as it attacked the body. In the late twentieth century, we have begun to realize that the way to approach disease is first to build up the strength of the body, the preventive aspect, and then also fight the microbe. In other words, it is no longer valuable simply to attack the disease without building up the strength of the immune system first.

YOUR IMMUNITY QUOTIENT — A TEST

At this point, it is of some use, both for learning about the immune system and for evaluating your own immune strengths, to move on to a simple test. The following quiz will give you a fairly good idea of your *Immunity Quotient,* or Im.Q. Admittedly, the rating scale is subjective; but the test scores will give you a quantitative method for estimating your general state of immunity. The total you achieve by adding up your scores from the individual "blocks" will give you an initial rating. But as you begin to incorporate more of this book's self-help hints, you will see your Im.Q. — and your immune function — improve. Retake this quiz at the end of one month and then at three-month intervals to reevaluate your Im.Q. and your resistance. At first, you may not understand all of the terms used or the reasoning behind the scores. As the book unfolds, each chapter will add to your understanding of the items scored in this test of your Immunity Quotient.

THE MASTER SHEET

(Mind/Body Connections)

Have not had a major illness in years. ✓	Have never suffered from allergies. ✓	Do not feel like an "outsider." ✓
10 pts.	9 pts.	8 pts.
Am generally confident. ✓	Cuts heal rapidly. ✓	Reasonably satisfied with career, income, or school.
7 pts.	6 pts.	5 pts.
Am not more than 10 lbs. over ideal weight. ✓	Have a circle of close friends. ✓	Readily get rid of rage, anger, hostility, and aggression. ✓
4 pts.	3 pts.	2 pts.

Your score _____54_____

Maximum score this block _____54_____

Drugs, Sex, and Intimacy Component

Do not use "hard" drugs, i.e., cocaine, heroin, amphetamine, etc. 10 pts.	Limit alcohol intake to 3 oz. per day or do not use it at all. 9 pts.	Do not smoke tobacco. 8 pts.
Have a satisfactory sex life (in *own* view). 7 pts.	Only one sex partner for a long period, or 6 pts.	Strictly limit sex partners. 5 pts.
Maintain and enjoy an intimate relationship. 4 pts.	Occasionally achieve an intimate relationship. 3 pts.	Rarely achieve intimacy. 2 pts.

Your score _____ 44 _____

Maximum score this block _____ 44 _____

Avoiding Unhealthy Food Component

Severely restrict fats and meats in diet. ✓ 10 pts.	Avoid smoked foods (containing nitrates, nitrites, and erythorbates). ✓ 9 pts.	Avoid food chemicals and additives (e.g., colorings and flavorings). ✓ 8 pts.
Avoid white and brown sugar. 7 pts.	Avoid refined white flour baked products. 6 pts.	Avoid deep-fried foods. ✓ 5 pts.
Avoid barbecued foods. 4 pts.	Avoid overeating. 3 pts.	Avoid or limit caffeine to 50 mg per day. ✓ 2 pts.

Your score _____ 34

Maximum score this block _____ 54

Healthful Food Component*

Eat high-fiber diet (e.g., more than 25 g per day).	Eat moderate-fiber diet (15 to 24 g per day).	Eat foods with anti-oxidants (e.g., fruits and vegetables rich in vitamins A, C, E, and selenium).
10 pts.	9 pts.	8 pts.
Eat seafood 3 times per week.	Eat whole-grain products.	Drink immune-stimu-lating herbal teas (Pau D'Arco, Mathake†).
7 pts.	6 pts.	5 pts.
Eat 25% of daily foods in raw state.	Eat chemical-free foods (i.e., organi-cally grown and pro-cessed).	Drink 8–16 oz. freshly squeezed juices (varied) daily.
4 pts.	3 pts.	2 pts.

Your score _____ 24 _____

Maximum score this block _____ 45 _____

* Score only one fiber cube, whichever is higher.
† Both kinds are particularly effective against candida infections.

Exercise Component: Choose One!

Exercise vigorously and completely* 7 times per week. *10 pts.*	Exercise vigorously and completely 6 times per week. *9 pts.*	Exercise vigorously and completely 5 times per week. *8 pts.*
Exercise vigorously and completely 4 times per week. ✓ *7 pts.*	Exercise vigorously and completely 3 times per week. *6 pts.*	Exercise vigorously and completely 2 times per week. *5 pts.*
Exercise vigorously and completely once per week. *4 pts.*	Exercise vigorously and completely occasionally. *3 pts.*	Beginning an exercise schedule. *2 pts.*

Your score _____ X

Maximum score this block _____ 10 _____

* ''Completely'' stands for the idea of balance in exercise and includes varied activities, stretching, breathing completely as in yoga, strength work as in weightlifting, maintaining aerobic capacity, etc.

The Vitamin and Mineral Component

Daily take:
beta-carotene
    (vitamin A) –
    15 mg (equiv.
    to 25,000 IU)
vitamin C – 2 g
vitamin E – 400 IU
selenium
multivitamin/mineral
    supplement.
 	
10 pts.
	Daily take
	    zinc supplement.
	
	9 pts.
		Daily take
		    calcium/magne-
		    sium supplement.
		
		8 pts.

Daily take
    vitamin B complex
    (50–100 mg).
 	
7 pts.
	Daily take
	    lecithin supple-
	    ment.
	
	6 pts.
		Daily take
		    pantothenic acid
		    and niacin supple-
		    ment.
		
		5 pts.

Daily take
    PABA (a subtle
    B vitamin)
    supplement.
 	
4 pts.
	Every other day take
	    vitamin C and
	    a multivitamin
	    (*without* iron).*
	
	3 pts.
		Every third or fourth
		    day take vitamin C
		    and a multivitamin
		    (*without* iron).*
		
		2 pts.

Your score _____

Maximum score this block _____ 49 _____

* Score one of last two cubes *only* when first 10-point maximum cube is unchecked.

WHAT IS YOUR IMMUNITY QUOTIENT?

Insert your scores from the building blocks you have just completed and compute your total score. Then, to see how you "rate," check the rating scale that follows.

Mind/Body Connections
Your score _____

Drugs, Sex, and Intimacy Component	Avoiding Unhealthy Food Component
Your score _____	Your score _____

Healthful Food Component	Exercise Component	The Vitamin and Mineral Component
Your score _____	Your score _____	Your score _____

Your total score _____

RATING YOUR IM.Q.

Scores between 230–256 = A+; 190–229 = A; 170–189 = B+; 150–169 = B; 140–149 = B–; 130–139 = Average; 120–129 = D; below 119 = F.

Although this is only a rough gauge of your immunity, it should begin to help you see the kinds of things that go into building a healthy immune system. For a medically accurate reading of your immune status, we suggest you see a physician, who can order the appropriate tests.

BUILDING MAXIMUM IMMUNITY

Influenza, cancer, herpes, candidiasis, various food and chemical allergies, rheumatoid arthritis, lupus, hepatitis, mononucleosis, malaria, and other disorders are all, to some degree, mediated by various aspects of the immune system. By learning how to stimulate the production of the essential immune fighters, the T and B cells — for example, by using specific nutrients — you can speed your own healing processes when ill or, better yet, prevent many serious problems, both infectious diseases and illnesses popularly thought to be of unknown origin. These and other healing connections are clearly stated in this book, with full references to the medical literature and instructions for increasing your immune competence.

We will begin by explaining in simple terms how the immune system works, both in minor disease — that is, in everyday operation — and under major stress, as in the face of a dangerous disease such as cancer. Then we will go on to give you specific hints and directions for improving your immunity. Finally, we will look at particular diseases and how they reflect impaired immunity, and how in most cases you can bolster your immune system against these devastating diseases. *Maximum Immunity* is not an either/or proposition alongside modern medicine. This book provides you with a common sense way to enhance your own natural resistance to illness — an approach that can work in conjunction with your physician's medical plan. *Maximum Immunity* will give you the information you need to take at least a part of your own health into your own hands. For instance, easily the most important single tool you have in bolstering your immune system is also the most obvious — your mind.

THE MIND: MASTER OF IMMUNITY

A sense of relative well-being, or of optimism, is essential to our resistance to infection, as well as to our overall state of health. But how this positive mental state is dependent upon the substrate of nutrients, degree of physical activity, even a sense of community (that is, within a circle of friends) is just beginning to be elucidated in the medical literature. We have all known that how we feel about our lives affects our physical health and that our physical state affects our feelings. These mind/body connections, mediated by the brain and its chemical messengers, are described throughout this book, giving you the simple "dos" and "don'ts" for maximum immunity.

"GENTLEMEN, GENTLEMEN, REMEMBER: MICROBES DO EXIST!"

When I was a young graduate student studying cell biology, I met a remarkable man — then and now a leading research psychologist. He convincingly demonstrated to me how powerful the emotions are in disease development and cure. As he cited case after case, I remember slowly losing my early resistance to the theory of psychosomatic causation. One case in particular I vividly recall — that of a banker in his mid-fifties dying of "incurable" leukemia. Through talk and understanding, my psychologist friend managed to get this dying man to share a lifelong secret — that ever since he was a little boy, he had dreamed of playing the violin and becoming a professional violinist. His stern father had ruled out this choice as being "too feminine"; consequently, a very unhappy banker was created. Then, at the "end" of his life, he took up the violin, and almost miraculously and against all the odds, the leukemia went into remission!

Delving into other such documented cases, I soon became so convinced of the mind's influence over the body that I was prepared to drop my studies and pursue psychology. Fortunately, my friend told me a story that kept me from changing *my* life. Upon receiving his doctoral degree, he and the other graduates were all loudly celebrating with one supportive case example after another at a kind of graduation celebration. The esteemed professor of the new science of psychosomatic medicine rose to the podium, silenced the celebrators, and said, "Gentlemen, gentlemen, you must remember, microbes do exist!"

Yes, microbes do exist, as do insects, allergies, harmful chemicals, radiation, the *lack* of protective nutrients, and inadequate physical stimulation. In this book, we hope to demonstrate the simple methods you can employ to maximize your ability to resist disease and recover more rapidly should you fall ill.

HOW DO WE KNOW IF VITAMINS AND MINERALS REALLY WORK TO STIMULATE IMMUNE FUNCTION?

The conventional medical establishment will tell you that vitamins do *not* work to protect you against immune disorders such as cancer. For example, a "major" study originally published in the journal *Cancer* purported to prove that taking vitamin A "pills" did not reduce the risk of developing cancer. This study was later quoted and requoted by other investigators (in other journals) who did not do their homework and check the original study. Let us go into this study for a moment.

The title of the study sounds authoritative: "Cancer Among Users of Preparations Containing Vitamin A: A Case-Control Investigation" (Smith and Jick 1978). These scientists interviewed 800 "newly diagnosed cancer patients and 3433 patients with certain non-malignant conditions" (as controls). The people interviewed for this study were asked only *if* they took vitamin A on a regular basis. *No attempt was made to determine the amount* (dosage) or *kind* of vitamin A in the "pills." With the right amount of vitamin A (more than 20,000 IU daily) from the best sources (fish liver oil or vegetables, not synthetic), there is a definite positive effect on the immune system. In Chapter 6, we report studies by medical researchers which support these immune-stimulating effects (for example, Chandra 1980; Neumann 1977; and Beisel et al. 1981).

The point we want to make here is that — despite the bias *against* the use of nutritional supplements by the conventional medical research establishment,* particularly those studies funded and reported by the American Cancer Society† — hun-

---

* The horizon holds promise, however. At a bastion of conventional therapy, the Sloan-Kettering Memorial Center in New York City, significant dosages of vitamin/mineral supplements are now routinely given in cancer therapy. Unfortunately, these are accompanied by radiation and chemotherapeutic agents, which effectively destroy immune response.

† The journal of this organization, *Cancer,* is supported in large part by the manufacturers of drugs used to treat cancer, or the associated pain. A recent issue of the journal contains a full-page ad that reads "Morphine: Pure and Simple." The medical establishment has not come very far in eighty years. This two-page display for morphine in a medical journal does not suggest a great deal of interest in preventive medicine.

dreds of positive studies and thousands of cured patients support this program for maximum immunity. While all the facts are not yet in, we must do what we have good reason to believe will help protect us against the immune disorders that threaten. By taking a positive approach through the measures outlined in this book, you can assert your own natural powers to protect yourself.

WHO SHOULD READ THIS BOOK?

Maximum Immunity is for anyone who would like to be healthy enough so that they won't become sick. If you are chronically ill and need help, you should read this book and apply our suggestions along with the recommendations made by your physician. If you have one of the immune diseases described in detail in Part III of this book, following the suggestions made here can help you strengthen your body's defenses against the illness. If you simply feel vulnerable, like everyone else in the world, you should read this book because, since you were born with the best immune system, the best resistance to illness, that anyone has yet invented, wouldn't it make sense to know how to build it and make it as strong as it can possibly be? And finally, you should read this book if you are healthy but are determined to stay that way, because this is a common sense, intelligent approach to developing your body's own internal resistance to illness.

We will begin by describing the components that make up your immune system and then providing examples of how they all work together to combat both simple and complex diseases. With that groundwork, we will give you the *facts* about how you can use psychology, nutrition, and exercise to strengthen your immunity. We will then talk about how major diseases disrupt the body's immune function and, finally, provide recommendations on how to live your life so as to minimize the potential for immune-related diseases.

○ 2 ○

What Is the Immune System?

SURVIVING IN A SEA OF ANTIGENS

"David" lived all his life in a specially controlled, germ-free environment in a hospital in Houston, Texas. Inside a plastic bubble, he breathed air filtered to remove any bacteria, viruses, or other foreign substances. His food was sterilized and introduced through air locks. Not until a bone marrow transplant at the age of twelve was he able to leave his bubble and feel for the first time his mother's kiss.

Through David's example, we all saw what it would mean to have an immune system that was not able to protect us from the billions of micro-organisms that exist unseen about us. David died at the age of twelve from complications following his unsuccessful bone marrow transplant — the longest any human had ever lived without a functioning immune system. Most children with such a severe immune problem succumb to massive infection before they are one year old.

But David's condition was a rare exception; most of us are able to move through the world and its countless invisible hazards without suffering constant illness.

Take "Alison," for example. As a nurse in the emergency room of a busy city hospital, she is exposed daily to a multitude of threats to her immune system. Sick patients in the waiting room sneeze, spreading viruses and bacteria through the air. Babies are brought in with measles, chicken pox, pneumonia, whooping cough, and other highly infectious diseases. Because Alison's hospital is in a port town, she also sees merchant seamen suffering from a bewildering variety of exotic tropical ailments. And yet Alison does not get sick any more often than her friends who work in the relative safety of offices downtown. In many different ways, her immune system is constantly vigilant, protecting her health.

"Howard" and "Vivian" are a healthy, active couple in their sixties. To celebrate Howard's retirement, they bought a mobile home and drove south into Mexico. During a stay at a seaside resort, they both ate seafood cocktails sold on the beach. As they continued on down the coast, Vivian began to feel weak and lose her appetite. Her skin took on a yellowish tinge, and her eyeballs became yellow. The obvious diagnosis: hepatitis. Howard, who had been in the military service in the tropics, had had hepatitis as a young man. He was unaffected by the hepatitis "bug" in Mexico; but Vivian's illness forced the couple to cut their trip short. After a recuperation period, she became well and also developed an immunity to hepatitis. In different ways, both Howard's and Vivian's immune systems defended them against the hepatitis virus.

Antigens. As these stories illustrate, our environment is filled with an astounding variety of things that have the capacity to make us sick. These "foreign agents" constantly trying to invade our bodies are known collectively as *antigens*. They include many different items: bacteria, viruses, fungi, dust, harmful chemicals, pollen grains, or proteins from food that has not been properly digested. Anything that triggers the immune system to respond is, by definition, an antigen.

Some antigens are not foreign agents at all but originate within our own bodies. Cancer cells, for example, are probably produced spontaneously in everyone's body, but in most people the immune system is able to identify and eliminate these cells before they grow out of control. Other antigens may not be so common, such as a transplanted kidney, or a blood transfusion of an incompatible blood type. In its attempt to protect the body against foreign invaders, the immune system may react against such well-intended materials, setting off reactions that can be disastrous.

A case in point was the heart from an ape transplanted into "Baby Fae." The hope of the physicians was that the baby's immature immune system would not reject the animal's heart the way a fully developed adult's certainly would, and that by using special immunosuppressive drugs, they could in effect trick the body into allowing the alien heart to work without interference. As it turned out, the baby did indeed survive almost twice as long as had been predicted (twelve days as opposed to six), but the side effect of the powerful immune system suppressing drugs was massive kidney failure, which was what caused her death.

Suppressing the immune system is not something that is done lightly. Many transplant patients die, not from the operation, but rather from pneumonia or other opportunistic infections that their bodies are unable to battle in their weakened state. Of particular concern is that immunosuppressive treatment seems to open the way for the development of cancer. There is an unusually high incidence of cancer among transplant patients who have received immune-suppressing drugs for a long time.

A case in point is a study of Kaposi's sarcoma in kidney transplant recipients conducted in Saudi Arabia (Akhtar 1984). Of the fifty-one kidney transplant patients who were followed over a seven-year period, four developed Kaposi's sarcoma! (Kaposi's sarcoma has recently received widespread publicity in the United States as one of the group of diseases involved in AIDS, or Acquired Immune Deficiency Syndrome.) While the exact cause of this disease is not certain, the high incidence in this Saudi group seems to confirm that immunosuppressive drugs employed in transplant surgery depress our bodily defenses so severely as to invite serious, often fatal, illnesses other than the one being treated.

THE MYSTERY OF IMMUNITY UNRAVELED

How are we able to survive in this sea of antigens — this swarm of invaders threatening from without, and from within? To be able to respond to all possible dangers, your immune system must be constantly on the alert, prepared to defend its territory — your body — against even the most unexpected threats, without exhausting its own resources in the process.

Preparedness for the unexpected. Your immune system must be able to deal with the antigens with which it has had no previous contact. Although it has the capacity to recognize and produce antibodies against some one million to one billion specific

antigens, the immune system can not foresee every possible antigen that might come along. Sooner or later, a completely new antigen will enter your body, and your immune system must be able
to combat it.

The influenza virus is an example. Actually, no such thing as
the flu virus exists; there are numerous varieties, and new ones
continue to evolve all the time. During the winter "flu season," we
often receive warning of a new strain of influenza. If our immune
systems did not have ways of dealing with these strange new viral
strains, we would be dying in huge numbers in flu epidemics. (Although the flu epidemic of 1918–1919 claimed some twenty million lives worldwide, the fatality rate since then has been only
about 1 percent.) Of course it takes a while for the immune system
to respond to the invading organism, and for some people with
weakened defenses, the battle can prove dangerous or even fatal.
But most of us are able to survive each new flu epidemic with no
worse than perhaps losing a few days from work.

Those who take vitamin C in large enough doses can often defeat the invading virus, as demonstrated by the twelve thousand
patients treated for flu and other viral infections by Robert F.
Cathcart III, M.D., of Los Altos, California. The specifics of the
right dosage and other self-protective maneuvers will be described
as we go along.

Distinguishing "foreign" from "self." Your immune system
must be able to react specifically to substances that are foreign in
origin and not a part of your body. It can tell the difference between "self" and "nonself" through a property known as *tolerance* — which means that it is able to ignore stimuli that are
constantly present, such as features of your body chemistry. In
much the same way, your nervous system ignores the sensation of
your clothes pressing against your skin or your hair touching the
back of your neck.

Sometimes tolerance works to our disadvantage, as when early
cancerous growths, perhaps disguised as part of the regular interior "landscape," are able to escape detection by the immune system. If they elude the immune defenses for long enough, such
tumors are able to become established and grow large.

While tolerance usually protects the body from attacking itself,
there are cases when tolerance breaks down. In the so-called *autoimmune diseases,* such as rheumatoid arthritis or lupus, the body's

immune defenses turn against the cells and tissues of the body they are designed to protect. Sometimes, also, the immune system's tendency to attack anything that is "nonself" has undesirable results — as when the body rejects a transplanted organ.

DIVERSITY OF RESPONSE

Viruses, bacteria, cancer cells, pollen, molds, and chemicals all have widely differing physical properties and many different ways of attacking the body and eluding the immune defenses. Your immune system must, therefore, have a variety of ways to ward off the attacks of these antigens and to overcome their defenses. Think again of Alison, the nurse in the emergency room. Each different micro-organism in the sneeze-laden air presents a different challenge to her immune system. To some of the disease organisms, Alison has already developed an immunity. Others must be dealt with as they present themselves, and viruses, bacteria, and molds are all handled differently.

The components of the immune system are organized and interconnected in such a way as to permit a remarkable flexibility of response. Rarely is your body limited to just one way of dealing with the challenge presented by an antigen. If one defense strategy does not work, your immune system is ready with another.

Adaptability. The immune system does not squander itself by maintaining large quantities of every weapon in readiness at all times. Rather, your body stores only a few of the fighting cells specifically matched to each possible invader. When a particular antigen presents itself, the cells specifically matched to it are stimulated to multiply into a whole army. In the case of Howard and Vivian on their Mexican vacation, Howard's immune system already contained some of the particular antibody needed to fend off the new invasion by the hepatitis virus, and it was prepared to make more rapidly. Vivian, on the other hand, did not have any specialized cells for this emergency, and so she experienced symptoms until her immune system was able to produce the kind of antibody needed to eliminate the invader.

The cells that make up the fighting forces of the immune system are essentially unspecialized. It is only when they reach the parts of the body where they come into contact with specific antigens that they receive their final programming and take on the characteristics needed to respond to the challenge. You can think of these fighting cells as recruits in boot camp, who must go through basic training before receiving their battle assignments.

While it is entertaining to think of the immune system as consisting of a lot of gallant little cells rushing around gobbling up invaders, there is much more to immunity than that. To explore the mystery of immunology, we will need to introduce a few technical terms. If you take the trouble now to grasp the basic principles, it will be much easier for you to understand the discussion later on how you can increase your own immunity. For a quick overview, the components of the immune system and their functions are highlighted in Table 1, at the end of this chapter.

YOUR BODY'S DEFENSE MECHANISM

As with so many of our bodily survival mechanisms, we take our immune system for granted. Just as you can not spend all your time making a conscious decision about when to inhale and when to exhale, you are not able to monitor every antigen that impinges on your body and then decide how to deal with it. Rather, it is your immune system — made up of specialized organs and cells under the overall supervision of your brain — that is programmed to take care of the day-to-day job of protecting you against foreign invaders.

Imagine that your body is a sovereign nation — a complete, separate organism living in a constantly changing environment. What prevents your body, the host country, from becoming a Petri dish for every kind of bacterium and virus? That is the job of your immune system. It is the immune system that protects you from attack by foreign and internal agents, that plans defensive actions, and that provides the necessary personnel and equipment. When the immune system is not functioning properly, it can mean disaster for the individual; if it fails to act, or if it acts inappropriately, the result can be serious illness or death.

THE DEFENSE CELLS

If you were to look at a drop of blood microscopically, you would see that more than 99 percent of the cells are red blood cells and the remaining 1 percent are white blood cells. (For a quick reference, a healthy adult shows about five million red cells and seven thousand white cells per cubic millimeter of blood sampled.) The white cells are different according to their function.* They are the main fighting troops of the immune system and are divided into three branches: *B cells, T cells,* and *macrophages.* Their job is to circulate through the blood and tissues to locate, trap, and destroy threatening invaders.

Both B and T cells (also called lymphocytes) begin their existence in the liver of about a nine-week-old fetus. They then migrate to the bone marrow, where they begin to follow different lines of development, specializing into varying kinds of "stem," or precursor, cells. The T cells then migrate from the bone marrow to the thymus gland, while the B cells remain in the bone marrow. This is why they are named as they are: the B cells for *bone marrow–derived* and the T cells for *thymus-derived.*

Not only do their histories differ, but the B and T cells also have distinct methods for dealing with antigens.

B cells. The B cells are responsible for producing *antibodies* — those substances specifically matched to each individual antigen and that help to neutralize or destroy that antigen.

When a B cell comes into contact with an antigen, it undergoes a physical change. It grows larger and divides into several cells, called *plasma cells,* which secrete the antibodies. Some of these antibodies then circulate throughout the body, where they can interact with the corresponding antigens. Others are secreted on the surface of B cells and help in recognizing antigens. It is because they release antibodies into the body fluids to combat antigens that the B cells are said to be involved in *humoral immunity.*

Another kind of B cell is the *memory cell,* which helps to develop a rapid antibody response to an antigen to which the body has been exposed in the past. This memory function is what protects you from diseases you had previously or for which you have received immunizations.

---

* White cells are grouped together as *leukocytes.* Only 25 to 30 percent of the total white cell count consists of *lymphocytes.* Not white cells per se; but part of this fighting system, are *plasma cells* and *macrophages.* To minimize confusion, I have used *lymphocyte* and *white blood cell* interchangeably, because *antibodies,* the most commonly understood term of immunity, result from interactions between plasma cells, macrophages, and these all-important lymphocytes.

T cells. T cells develop into various specialized kinds of cells responsible for *cell-mediated* immune reactions — which means that rather than responding to the presence of antigens by producing antibodies, they influence neighboring white blood cells and other cells. T cells are effective at fighting bacteria, fungi, parasites, and intracellular viruses (those viruses that attack from within the body's cells).

"On" and "off" with helpers and suppressors. Some T cells influence other cells by turning on or off reactions in the immune system. *T helper cells* may induce B cells to respond to the presence of an antigen, and they may also stimulate activity in other T cells. *T suppressor cells* operate in the opposite direction, regulating the immune response by "turning off" certain cell activity. For example, T suppressor cells may interfere with T helper cells or inhibit B cells from producing antibodies.

You may wonder why the immune system must include these two opposing forms of T cells. The T helpers and T suppressors help to maintain a delicate balance in the immune response. If the balance is disturbed, you lose your protection against foreign and internal antigens. In fact, the ratio of T helpers to T suppressors is considered an indicator of the general state of the immune system. The normal condition is a ratio of approximately 1.8 helpers to each suppressor (1.8:1). Ratios that are either markedly higher or lower indicate immune malfunction.

For example, patients with AIDS often have a ratio of 1:1 or less. Here the number of T suppressor cells has risen to such an extent that these "off" switch cells actually destroy the body's natural immunity. Other examples of diseases with abnormal helper to suppressor ratios are listed in Appendix 1.

Other kinds of T cells may react with antigens without the involvement of B cells. *Natural killer cells* (NK cells) are able to kill foreign cells through direct contact, by producing a *cytotoxin,* or cell poison. NK cells are believed to be a form of T cell (Fox 1981). A fascinating aspect of these defensive cells is that they are triggered to kill invaders without any known antigenic stimulation and without any antibody to the invader being released.

The B and T cells in the thymus and bone marrow are essentially unspecialized, receiving their final programming when they reach the areas where they come into contact with antigens. For example, once they have identified an antigen, the T cells may in-

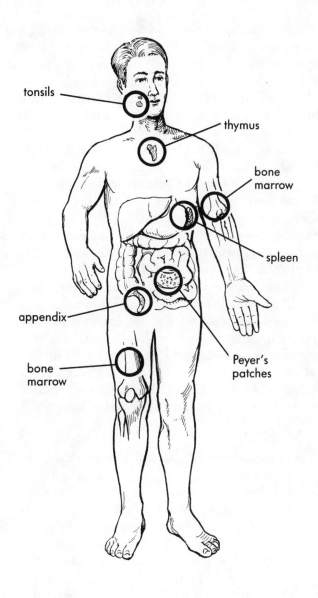

tonsils

thymus

bone
marrow

spleen

appendix

Peyer's
patches

bone
marrow

Fig. 1. ORGANS OF THE IMMUNE SYSTEM
(Lymph nodes not shown)

fluence what antibodies are produced in the developing B cells. Once the correct antibody is selected, it is rapidly produced, perhaps rising in that area to a level more than one thousand times normal. Of course, once the threatening substance has been eliminated, the antibody level must return to normal. This is where the T suppressor cells play their part, turning off the immune response to that antigen.

Macrophages. The B and T cells interact not only with each other, but also with the other major fighting cells in the immune system — the macrophages. These are large white blood cells produced in the bone marrow along with the B cells, the T cell precursors, and the red blood cells.

Macrophages are called into play once an antigen has been recognized. Like microscopic "Pac-Men," the macrophages have the function of gobbling up antigens. The scientific term for this consumption of antigens is *phagocytosis,* and all the types of cells that engage in phagocytosis are known as *phagocytes.*

Macrophages can fight antigens in different ways. The macrophage may engulf an antigen without identifying it as a foreign particle and process it so that it is easier for white cells to recognize it as an invader. Once the antigen is identified, it is attacked; then the macrophages break up the entire antigen-antibody complex, eventually excreting the invader from the body.

OVERALL COMMAND: THE LYMPHATIC SYSTEM

If the macrophages and the B and T cells are somewhat akin to the troops in a combat situation, then the lymphatic system can be considered their command. (As we will see in Chapter 4, the brain is the center of all decision making and can be made to control aspects of immune functioning, even the lymph cells.)

The *lymphatic system* is another name for all the organs of the immune system and is made up of two subdivisions: *primary* (or central) and *secondary* (or peripheral) organs. The primary organs of immunity are the *thymus* and *bone marrow;* the secondary organs include the *lymph nodes, spleen, tonsils, appendix, Peyer's patches,* and small *specialized* lymph *nodules* in the membranes of the intestines.

The fighting cells of immunity are *produced* in the primary organs, but do not actually come into contact with foreign invaders until they reach the secondary organs, where they initiate their defensive response.

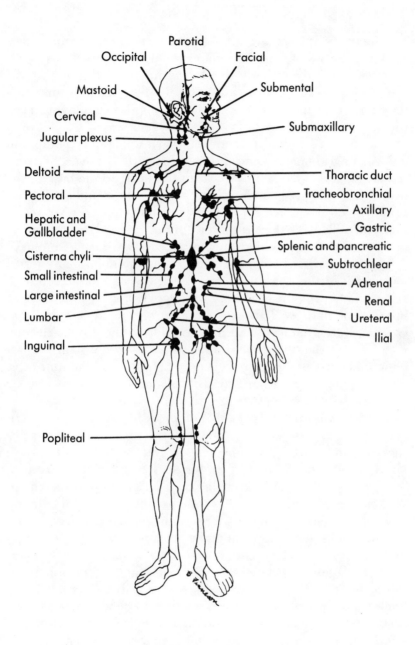

Fig. 2. LYMPH NODES OF THE BODY
(Source: Kimber et al. 1966)

Primary lymphatic organs. The thymus is one of your body's more mysterious organs. This gland in the chest reaches its maximum size, relative to body weight, during early childhood, and then begins to shrink in relative size. Its function was unknown for many years, but now the thymus is recognized as playing a key role in maintaining the body's immune defenses.

You can get an idea of where your thymus gland is by tapping on your breastbone; it is located deep beneath this bone, between the lungs, and extends upward from the heart to the base of the neck.* The thymus gland is shaped like a pyramid and is made up of many lobules. Each lobe consists of an outer cortex and an inner medulla. The T cells mature in the cortex, later migrating into the medulla of the thymus gland for release during an illness.

The *bone marrow* is the soft material in the hollow interior of long bones of the arms and legs. As already stated, the B and T cells, after leaving the fetal liver, undergo their early development in the bone marrow. It is here also that red blood cells and macrophages are produced. You may recall from the story of the boy who lived in the bubble that a bone marrow transplant was attempted in order to give him a supply of functional immune cells. Normally functioning bone marrow is a crucial element of your immune defenses.

Secondary lymphatic organs. You probably know from experience where at least some of your lymph nodes are located, since these organs tend to become tender and swollen with certain kinds of infection. This is why your doctor feels your neck, armpits, and groin when you go in for a checkup — to search for swollen lymph areas. These pea-shaped organs are also found along the spine, near the heart, around the digestive organs, and in the membranes supporting the intestinal tract. The lymph nodes are connected by a network of vessels that receive drainage from the organs associated with the nodes and from throughout the body. This *lymphatic duct system* serves as both the *information network* and the *transportation complex* for your body's defense personnel. In areas where there is no direct lymphatic drainage, lymphatic materials are transported by the blood. The lymph nodes

---

* The dish known as "sweetbreads" is made from the thymus of a cow.

contain specialized compartments — some containing B cells, some with T cells, and some containing macrophages. Webbed areas in the lymph nodes trap antigens and filter them out of the clear lymphatic fluid, or lymph.

The *spleen* is a spongy organ located in the left side of the abdominal cavity between the stomach, the left kidney, and the ribs. The blood carries B cells, T cells, antigens, macrophages, and antigen-reactive cells to the spleen, which supports their interactions — helping in the production of antibodies, the maintenance of cellular immunity, and the recirculation of white cells. In the past, it was fashionable for doctors to remove the spleen when they were operating on something else, since spleen removal did not seem to do any obvious harm. Fortunately, doctors today are more reluctant to remove an organ — especially one so integral to the immune system — simply because the abdomen is open. We now know that people whose spleens have been damaged by injury or disease have a greatly increased susceptibility to infection.

The *tonsils* are complexes of lymphoid tissues, much like lymph nodes, situated in several different locations in the throat. Like the lymph nodes, the tonsils contain B and T cells; and like the spleen, the tonsils were at one time removed at the slightest provocation. For many generations of children, "having their tonsils out" was their first and only hospital experience. Tonsillectomy is still one of the most frequently performed operations, but the rate has been dropping rapidly. Even so, most of the tonsillectomies performed are probably not necessary. The fact that the tonsils become swollen and inflamed indicates that they are doing their job — not that they should be removed.

The tonsillectomy is but one example of "fad" surgery. At the turn of the century, wealthy English people often elected to have their colons removed in what was then a fad surgical procedure termed colectomy. This was thought somehow beneficial. While the meticulous by-passed their animal heritage, defecating in little rubber bags (!), there was and is no scientific evidence to support the value of such a procedure.

Today, coronary by-pass surgery is the rage. Unfortunately, the five-year survival rates are about equal among those people with angina who elect this surgery and those who do not.

The appendix, Peyer's patches, and intestinal nodes are small components of the lymphatic drainage system. They are primarily locations where B cells mature and where antibodies are produced in the intestinal region. The appendix has gained a notoriety far beyond its functional significance as yet another popular candidate for surgical removal. For reasons not entirely clear (but which may be connected to low-fiber, high-sugar diets), the appendix has a distressing tendency to become inflamed and to threaten rupture. Supporting the belief that most appendectomies are unnecessary is the fact that in China 90 percent of twenty thousand patients with acute appendicitis were treated by *nonsurgical* means (using herbal drugs) with total success or "uneventful recovery" (NAS 1975).

These, then, are the cells and organs that play the leading roles in the lifelong drama of your immune defense system. How they all work together to battle specific antigens on the molecular level is the subject of the next chapter.

TABLE I

Elements of the Immune System

Name	Location	Function
B Cells	Mature in bone marrow and circulate throughout body.	Humoral immunity: responsible for producing antibodies that promote immunity against bacteria and viruses.
Plasma cells	Throughout body.	Stimulated B cells mature into plasma cells, which are antibody factories.
Memory cells	Throughout body.	Other cells into which some B cells mature. These help develop rapid antibody response to antigens to which the host has previously been exposed.
T Cells	Mature in thymus gland and circulate throughout body.	Cell-mediated immunity: influence certain white and other cells to combat antigens; also fight antigens directly. Involved in transplant and tumor immunity; also viral, mycobacterial, fungal, and protozoal immunity.
T helper cells	Throughout body.	Stimulate B cells and other T cells to respond to the presence of an antigen.

Name	Location	Function
T suppressor cells	Throughout body.	Regulatory inhibitors of immune response. Prevent B cells from being stimulated by antigen, and suppress helper T cell response, keeping immune response in balance.
Natural killer cells	Throughout body.	T cell derived white cells that kill foreign cells directly, by producing cytotoxin.
Macrophages	Produced in bone marrow and circulate throughout body.	Phagocytize (engulf and digest) antigens; process antigens for easier recognition by T cells.
Antibodies (=IgG, IgA, IgM, IgD, IgE — see Chapter 3)	Produced by B cells and circulate throughout body. (Found in the gamma globulin portion of the plasma proteins.)	Fight antigens by combining with the specific antigen that stimulated their production; disable bacteria from producing toxins, coat antigens for consumption by scavenger cells, block viruses from entering body cells.
Complement (see Chapter 4)	Throughout body.	Series of some 20 proteins with enzyme activity, which augment antigen-antibody reactions. Involved in inflammatory reaction and in combating micro-organisms.
Thymus	Upper chest.	Site of T cell maturation.
Bone marrow	Long bones of arms and legs.	Site of early development of B and T cells and of B cell maturation; also site of production of macrophages.
Lymph nodes	Neck, armpits, groin, along spine, near heart, around digestive organs.	Sites of B and T cell activity and filtration of lymph to remove antigens.
Spleen	Left side of abdomen.	Site of interaction of B cells, T cells, antigens, macrophages, and antigen-reactive cells.
Tonsils	Throat.	Site of T and B cell activity.
Appendix, Peyer's patches, intestinal nodules	Intestinal region.	Sites of B cell maturation and antibody production.
Interferons (see Chapter 4)	Infected cells.	The first line of defense against invading viruses, they are proteins made by our cells under viral attack and serve to inhibit the multiplication of a broad range of viruses.

· 3 ·

How Immunity
Works

WHAT HAPPENS WHEN WE GET SICK?

When our resistance is "down" or we are exposed to an inordinate number of disease organisms (antigens), we become ill. Here is what happens. During the first phase of infection, white blood cells attack the invaders at the site of infection, engulfing the antigens and breaking them apart. The first line of white cells is then followed by a second line of white cells that engulfs both the offending *and* defending cells, removing them from the site of infection, to eliminate the toxins or other harmful substances.

During this battle, the blood supply to the digestive system is reduced — which is why we lose our appetite. Our temperature rises; we call it a fever. These changes are necessary to speed up the chemical reactions required for our recovery. So much intense energy is expended on an invisible, cellular level, that little energy is left for muscular action. The reason we cannot think too clearly during this phase of the battle is that the brain is confused by poisons in the blood, resulting from the destroyed invaders, as well as by the elevated temperature.

When the infection is controlled, the macrophages return to the lymphoid tissue, carrying with them particles of the destroyed antigen. Future defense cells result from these macrophages. Because they contain portions of the invaders, a later infection by the same invaders is immediately recognized by the defending cells.

WHAT ANTIGENS ARE MADE OF

All of our "enemies," or antigens, have a distinctive chemical composition that contains protein, and every protein is made up of "building blocks" of amino acids, arranged in a precise sequence. This chemical structure causes the antigens to fold at various points, creating a unique three-dimensional shape. It is this unique shape of the attacking antigen that allows a defending antibody to recognize it.

ANTIBODIES, OR IG'S

Antibodies are also made up of proteins. Your immune system has evolved five types of antibodies, each having different structures and performing different functions. The abbreviation for these different antibodies is *Ig* (short for *immunoglobulins,* or small, round bodies of immunity). The five types of antibodies are known by their initials: IgG, IgA, IgM, IgD, and IgE. The most common of these is IgG, which makes up about 70 percent of the antibodies contained in tissues. Table 2 gives you a quick reference to each of these types of antibodies and what they do.

All the antibody structures contain Y shapes. It is the upper, branching portion of the Y that differs among the various types of antibodies. This difference in shape is due to the varying chain of amino acids in each antibody. And, the differing shapes enable antibodies to recognize, lock on to, and destroy an invading antigen.

Lock and key. The exposed surface of each antigen has distinctive physical and chemical features that are recognized by the antibodies as *combining sites.* The Y-shaped top of the antibody fits the exposed combining site of the antigen like an intricate, three-dimensional lock and key. Since there are two branches to the Y, there are two specific combining sites on each antibody. In an actual situation in the body, one antigen cell might be surrounded by a swarm of antibodies, each attached to a pair of combining sites on the antigen's surface.

Immune memory. Once your body has been exposed to a particular antigen and survived the attack, your immune system has a "memory" of that antigen. This long-term memory is an important feature of immune functioning. You may not be exposed to the same antigen for years after the first attack, but whenever you encounter that antigen again, your immune system will be ready for it, and the antigen will be rapidly taken care of.

Your first bout with a disease may make you quite sick, because it takes a while for your immune system to marshal its forces against the invader. For example, if you had measles as a child, you most likely had a fever as well as a skin rash and felt miserable for a few days. Once you got out of school, you might not have been exposed to a measles virus for years — especially since the measles vaccine has greatly reduced the incidence of this disease in recent years. Then perhaps your own child brought the "bug" home from school. This time you had the antibody required to combat the virus and did not get sick at all, although your youngster, if not vaccinated, may have gone through several days of being ill.

Vaccination. The long-term memory of the immune system is the feature put to use in vaccination, which is the injection into

TABLE 2

Types of Antibodies

Antibody	Function
IgG	Most common. Major Ig in defense against microbes. Coats micro-organisms, speeding their destruction by other immune system cells. Confers long-standing immunity.
IgM	Major Ig produced in primary antibody response. Circulates in the blood stream, where it kills bacteria. Increases during acute stage of an infection. Usually forms in star-shaped clusters.
IgA	Concentrates in body fluids (tears; saliva; respiratory, genitourinary, and gastrointestinal secretions) guarding body entrances. First line of defense against invading pathogens and food allergens. Major Ig in defense against viruses.
IgE	Involved in allergic reactions. Attaches to surface of mast cell,* and on encountering its matching antigen, stimulates the mast cell to pour out its contents. Also fights parasites.
IgD	Major Ig present on surface of B cells; may be involved in differentiation of these cells.

*Mast cells are found in connective tissue. They are numerous along blood vessel beds, form the anticoagulant heparin, and release histamine in allergic and inflammatory reactions.

the body of a weakened or dead strain of an antigen. The antigen in a vaccine acts the same way as the measles virus did on your first exposure to it, although without producing a full-blown illness. The immune system identifies the antigen in the vaccine, remembers it, and repels any future attacks by that particular antigen. Just how the immune system is able to "remember" a particular antigen is not fully understood; it is likely that minute amounts of the antigen are kept in the system to serve as a reminder.

The modern use of vaccination dates back to the English physician Edward Jenner, who in 1796 introduced the administration of a small dose of cowpox to humans, with the intent of creating immunity to smallpox. Centuries before Jenner, ancient Chinese and Arabic physicians succeeded in inducing immunity by deliberately transmitting smallpox to healthy persons via inhalation of powdered smallpox crusts from diseased people. In fact, wealthy Chinese sometimes carried "old" smallpox growths on their travels, distributing them to relatives as a token of their good wishes!

At one time, smallpox was a dreaded scourge, exterminating whole groups of humans. When Europeans brought smallpox to the New World from Europe, entire Indian tribes were annihilated by the disease. This was repeated in the South Seas, where nations of healthy people without previous immunity to the smallpox virus rapidly succumbed to the disease.

Eventually, through a worldwide vaccination campaign, smallpox became the first human disease to be almost completely eradicated. The last *naturally* acquired case (as opposed to laboratory contamination) of smallpox was reported in Somalia in 1977. Since then, there have been few cases of smallpox in the world, and vaccination is no longer routinely performed. Besides smallpox, a number of other formerly dread killing and crippling diseases, including diphtheria, polio, and even measles, have been effectively eradicated in the United States due to an aggressive program of vaccination (or immunization). Such immunization programs are not without their risks, however. Later in this book, we will examine the current controversy over DPT shots and other forms of immunization.

Your antibody heritage. Since antibodies are produced by the B cells, they trace their origins back to the fetal liver. How much did your parents contribute to your original store of antibodies?

According to the so-called *germline theory*, an infant inherits *all* of its antibodies genetically, from the parents. According to another theory, the *somatic mutation theory*, the mother passes on only a few antibodies — genetically through the placenta, as well as through her milk — which then mutate into all the rest. This theory thus constitutes a strong argument for the benefits of breast-feeding. In fact, the evidence is solid that breast-fed infants have fewer illnesses (infections, allergies, etc.) than those who are bottle fed.

The superior nutritional value of human milk for human infants explains this protective value in part, but *colostrum* contains life-saving antibodies that are not found in cow, goat, or soy milk.

"Sins of the mothers." Natural immunity really does begin at birth. When you consider that many diseases (syphilis, herpes, etc.) can be transmitted from mother to child in the birth canal, and that drugs and chemicals (including alcohol, tobacco, caffeine, and even artificial sweeteners) cross the placenta, you can see why so much of who we become depends upon who our mother was, how she cared for herself during gestation and nursing, and how she fed us when we were children.

Obvious as this might be, it bears repeating. As the philosopher Lao-tzu wrote thousands of years ago, "Nature is extremely impartial." It may be an unequal burden that falls upon women, but it has profound consequences. Seen from this perspective, human existence logically proceeds beyond the "sins-of-the-fathers" moralism, following laws related instead to the "sins of the mothers."

Earning your immunity. But "fate" is not irrevocable. The entire purpose of this book is to demonstrate what you can do to bolster, even surpass, your "inherited" level of immunity. In the case of your antibody stores, we have seen that no matter how antibodies are acquired in the first place, your immune system acquires others later in life. This can be done *actively*, with the immune system developing antibodies using its own resources. For example, when your immune system encounters a new antigen, it is usually able to synthesize a new antibody (or a modified form of an existing antibody) specifically matched to that antigen. This process is going on all the time in your body.

It is also possible for you to acquire antibodies *passively*. This is not the same as vaccination. In this case, antibody is extracted from a person who has already had the disease in question (or been vaccinated for it) and introduced into another person. The recipient is then able to use this passively acquired antibody as his own.

As an example of the difference between active and passive immunity, recall the story of the elderly couple at the beginning of the last chapter who were exposed to hepatitis on their vacation. Howard had acquired his immunity to hepatitis actively, years earlier, through exposure to the disease. Passive immunity to hepatitis can be acquired through injections of *gamma globulin,* a concentrated form of antibodies. If Vivian had gotten a gamma globulin shot before traveling to Mexico, her symptoms would not have been so severe when she contracted the disease. (Gamma globulin does not *prevent* infection from hepatitis, but does help to minimize the symptoms.)

WHY DO WE GET SICK?

With such a complex and impressive system of immune defenses, you may wonder why people ever get sick. The reason is that there is a time lapse between the moment a foreign agent enters the body and when the immune system finally destroys it. In the interim, the pathogen (disease-producing organism) is doing its damage to the body — killing cells, making toxins, devouring nutrients and energy. Once the immune system has the intruder under control, it still takes a while for the body to repair itself. The severity and duration of the attack determines how long the body will need to recuperate.

Now that you have an overview of the immune system, and some familiarity with the terms used to describe what goes on at the cellular level, you are ready to understand how to maintain and stimulate your immune system.

In Part II, you will find a three-tiered approach for achieving and maintaining maximum immunity — how to control and coordinate mind, diet, and exercise in a unified plan, based on solid, scientific evidence.

PART II

BUILDING IMMUNITY

Overview

A UNIFIED IMMUNITY PROGRAM

Now that we know that there is more to immunity than how white blood cells combat threatening microbes, we can use the following three-tiered approach to immunological health.

Knowing *what* the immune system consists of, *how* it maintains surveillance, and *when* its cells go into action will help us unify psychology (mind), biochemistry (diet), and physiology (exercise).

Obviously, we all eat, walk, and try to will ourselves healthy to some degree. Beyond that, even popping a multivitamin, jogging, and using one of the meditation or prayer-based "mind" methods is not adequate for the stresses of contemporary existence. As we approach our thirties, we notice certain changes — maybe more colds, less energy, a tendency to gain weight, decreased sexual strength, and so on. This is generally thought to be a "natural," "slowing-down" process, but it can be overcome.

Have you ever noticed the supervital fifty-year-old who runs rings around younger acquaintances? Or the octogenarian with wit and energy? Each of them has a secret. It may not be based on the three-tiered program described in this book, but if you get to know these vital people, you will likely discover that they follow an orderly, rational approach to surviving and thriving in a disorderly world.

Many people like to tell a story about a relative who lived into the eighties or nineties without paying any obvious attention to health. Some relish boasting of the ninety-year-old uncle who drank glasses of whiskey and smoked five cigars each day. Perhaps there are such people, but they are the exceptions, the immunological rogues. Most of us need strong controls to survive, even stronger direction to thrive. We have seen this in school, in our careers, in sports, and within our families. Those who applied themselves, early on, to a rigorous system of achievement generally went further than those who ignored all direction, were lazy, or followed a helter-skelter program.

The same is true with immunological health. It does not come naturally, but must be worked at. Learning how to control our bladder and our bowel, being fed nutritious foods, being cleaned and loved are all early elements of immunological training. As we get older and learn more about how to care for ourselves, a pattern of cause and effect begins to come clear to us. If we abuse our health by indulging in sweets or alcohol, headaches and other minor upsets follow. When we manage to follow a reasonable plan of diet and exercise, we feel stronger and more able to handle our challenges.

But most of us reach a point, usually in adolescence, when we think we are doing well enough, and we cease to investigate any more about health maintenance. Then, about twenty years later, perhaps in our thirties or forties, we begin to worry about getting sick and dying prematurely. This is the time to sharply analyze what we are doing and integrate the disparate elements of health we have begun to follow.

In the section that follows we will see how mind, matter, and motion can be unified to maintain maximum immunity.

∘ 4 ∘

The Psychology of Immunity

OR MIND OVER MICROBES

THE RELATIONSHIP BETWEEN medicine and behavior has come of age. What was once largely anecdotal has now emerged as a science. Now we are able to see, with a great deal of certainty, how mood or mind affects the disease or health processes, and how to resist succumbing to illness when stress or other behavioral factors threaten to overwhelm our innate defenses.

The executive who jogs before work and meditates after meetings, the athlete who disavows overly rich meals, the entertainer who does not use alcohol but relies instead on biofeedback techniques to restore equilibrium are examples of dramatic social changes. They contrast the martini lunch, the steak and eggs breakfast, the hard drinking nights of a decade or so ago.

A leader in the new field of *psychoneuroimmunology* who has generated excitement by his findings defines disease as "any persistent harmful disturbance of its equilibrium" (Cunningham 1981). This breaking field has led to new understanding of the relationships among three subsystems that maintain this equilibrium. These interrelating systems are known as the *nervous* (i.e., brain and spinal cord), *endocrine* (i.e., hormones), and *immune* systems.

On another level, the interconnections between "social, psychological, and somatic events" are what this fascinating field is all about, according to Professor Cunningham. As we develop "mental and immune memory," exchanges take place that make us sick if we fail to adapt adequately or help us to maintain our strength if our adaptations are right.

Going beyond our present knowledge of the healing value of rest and psychological support, the findings of this "explosive" field can now help us face the minefields of life, bringing us perhaps to the level of control demonstrated by mystics.

By learning how to control our mind, subtle hormonal changes emerge that then control our biochemical reality. This is the promise — the chapter offers you a way to begin fulfilling that promise.

MIND, BODY, AND IMMUNITY

Sometimes we need to come the long way around to rediscover ancient folk wisdom. Our great-grandmothers would not have been the least bit surprised to learn that depression or a stressful life change could lead to illness. But as the science of immunology began to uncover the incredibly complex interactions of our body's billions of defense cells, the role of the mind dropped out of the picture. Scientists began to think of our immune defenses as a self-contained system that responded automatically to the stimulus of an antigen. It seemed as if the nervous system was not necessary to the operation of our intricate immune mechanisms.

Now we know that things are not that clear cut. Our great-grandmothers were right: it is now evident that attitudes, beliefs, and emotions *can* influence immunity, and that the immune system can even be *conditioned* — tricked into responding by psychological devices.

The mind and body interact in many ways to influence immunity. Psychological stress releases powerful hormones that suppress our immune defenses; and our susceptibility to many diseases, from the common cold to cancer, is partly a function of how well we handle stressful situations. Eating the proper diet not only nourishes our immune system directly, but it also strengthens our psychological health, and thus helps us to manage stress and heal ourselves more effectively. Exercise also creates a positive psychological state that is immunity enhancing. Managing stress, both through restructuring false beliefs and by learning relaxation techniques, can greatly reduce our susceptibility to illness.

And if you *do* get sick, a positive, optimistic attitude, or the psychological support of a group of fellow patients, can be one of the most important factors in your cure.

This is why many of the items on the Master Sheet (Mind/Body Connections) in the Im.Q. quiz in Chapter 1 were concerned with psychological factors. A sense of belonging, confidence, life satisfaction, friendships, and the ability to let go of negative feelings correlate closely with strong immune defenses, good physical health, and long life. And the best news of all is that these psychological factors are generally under your control!

In this chapter we will examine the evidence indicating that psychological factors influence immunity, as well as show the many ways in which you can use the powers of your own mind to increase your immune defenses.

STRESS AND CORTISOL

Dozens of times, we have all seen how stress can lead to illness: a young salesman loses an important account and suffers a recurrence of herpes; a college woman at the end of exams comes down with the flu; a mother, shortly after the last of her children leaves home, develops breast cancer. Despite such examples from everyday experience, medical science has been slow to discover just how the mind influences the immune system. The story begins back in the 1930s with the recognition of *the stress response.*

The stress response. There are many parallels between the nervous system and the immune system. Although they operate in entirely different ways, both receive information from outside and inside the body, process it, and produce adaptive responses to these stimuli. In the case of the immune system, the typical stimulus is an antigen; in the nervous system it is a *stressor,* or stress-producing event. The immune system responds with a complex immune response; for the nervous system, the adaptive response is the stress response.

Hans Selye, an early pioneer in stress research, first defined stress in 1936 as a nonspecific response by the body to any demand made upon it to readjust. It did not matter what the stimulus, or stressor, was; as long as it was sufficiently strong, the same response would apply. When Selye first observed the effects of stress in animals, he discovered a characteristic three-part set of physiological changes: enlargement of the adrenal cortex; intense atrophy of the thymus, spleen, and lymph nodes; and deep, bleeding stomach and duodenal ulcers. The immune system, as represented by the thymus, spleen, and lymph nodes, was obviously intimately involved in the stress response.

According to Selye, the potent hormones released by the stress response can damage the body's organs, the nervous system, and the immune mechanisms. The stress response begins in the brain in a small area known as the *hypothalamus,* which responds to stress by triggering the *pituitary* gland to release hormones that govern the body's endocrine system. As a result, the medulla, or inner part, of the *adrenal* glands releases the hormone *adrenalin;* and the cortex, or outer part of the adrenals, releases a group of hormones called *corticosteroids.*

Adrenalin is easy to feel. You are very familiar with the "adrenalin rush" that occurs in a threatening situation, such as when you swerve to avoid a collision while driving. Adrenalin is what mobilizes your body for rapid response to perceived danger. It can also trigger the release of other hormones to speed metabolism.

The other stress-related hormones, the corticosteroids, cannot be felt directly, but they have a telling and wide-ranging effect on your immune system. It is the chronic secretion of these hormones that is suspected to cause the major damage in stress-related diseases.

Cortisol in stress-related diseases. There is strong evidence that a common denominator in many stress-related diseases is an elevated level of *cortisol* in the blood. Cortisol is another name for *hydrocortisone,* one of the corticosteroids secreted by the adrenal cortex. Chronically elevated cortisol levels, resulting from unrelieved stress, may actually be the cause, or a cause, of chronic diseases.

Cortisol is known to be a powerful immunosuppressant. It breaks down lymphoid tissues in the thymus and lymph nodes, reduces the level of T helper cells and increases T suppressors, and inhibits the production of natural killer cells. Cortisol also reduces virus-fighting *interferon* (Fauman 1982; Sapse 1984). Interferon is a naturally occurring antiviral agent, one produced by the body as a first line of defense against invading viruses. It was first discovered in 1957 and found able to inhibit most viruses. This led researchers to believe they could synthesize interferon-like drugs, which would become as useful as antibiotics. Unfortunately the chemical agents they selected to induce interferon production within the body proved to be highly toxic. Scientists then tried to coax white blood cells to produce interferon, which was far safer and more effective.

While genetic engineers compete to produce interferon in their high-technology laboratories and market it at astronomical prices, the human body may prove to be the best place to stimulate production of this substance. Based upon clinical results with many thousands of cases, several prominent physicians (described later, in Chapters 6 and 10) who have successfully treated a wide spectrum of viral illnesses with vitamin C and other nutrients believe that these "antiviral vitamins" work by stimulating the body to produce interferon.

But, we should return to our main point, cortisol. A wide range of diseases are associated with elevated cortisol levels, including depression, cancer, hypertension, ulcers, heart attack, diabetes, infections, alcoholism, obesity, arthritis, stroke, psychoses of the aging, skin diseases, Parkinson's disease, multiple sclerosis, myasthenia gravis, and even perhaps Alzheimer's disease. Elevated levels of cortisol are even reported to be a useful predictor of suicide (Sapse 1984).

Serious problems sometimes occur in patients who are treated with corticosteroid drugs. These drugs are used to treat a number of diseases, including rheumatoid arthritis, kidney disease, and leukemia. When corticosteroids are used therapeutically, cortisol levels rise, often inducing conditions that mimic other chronic diseases, such as diabetes, hypertension, and various mental disturbances. When the drugs are discontinued, such symptoms disappear.

Cortisol-lowering substances. A number of substances have been observed to produce dramatic, often unexpected improvements in various chronic diseases. These chronic diseases have little in common except the fact that they are all marked by elevated cortisol levels. The pharmaceuticals in question all have the ability to lower blood cortisol levels, which apparently accounts for their success in improving symptoms (Sapse 1984). Descriptions of these cortisol-lowering substances follow.

Dilantin, also known as phenytoin sodium or diphenylhydan-toin sodium, is a drug used to treat epilepsy. This drug received widespread attention through Jack Dreyfus's book, *A Remarkable Medicine Has Been Overlooked* (1982). Dreyfus, a wealthy financier, spent a fortune to report that Dilantin was beneficial in a wide range of diseases including depression, hypertension, ulcers, migraine headaches, and many others. According to research reports, Dilantin has cortisol-antagonistic abilities.

Procaine hydrochloride, the generic name for the anesthetic Novocain, is an ingredient in the controversial "anti-aging" drug Gerovital H_3. Procaine has reportedly been able to prevent ulcers from being induced experimentally by stress in animals. Procaine's anticortisol effects may explain some of its reported beneficial effects in people who take it to forestall the ravages of aging.

Vitamin C, or ascorbic acid, is a very important vitamin that inhibits cortisol following adrenal stimulation. Of all the cortisol-lowering substances in this list, vitamin C is by far the safest to use. Its cortisol-lowering properties may be at least partly responsible for its helpful effects in treating viral diseases.

Aspirin, chemically composed of salicylates, is known to reduce cortisol levels, even when these levels are normal.

Cimetidine, also known by the brand name Tagamet, is a new class of drug used in the treatment of ulcers. In rats cimetidine prevented the development of gastric ulcers from being induced by the chronic administration of corticosteroids.

Kronos is an experimental version of the anesthetic and heart drug lidocaine. Kronos was developed specifically with the cortisol theory in mind and may prove to be the first of a new class of drugs known as *cortisol antagonists.*

Cortisol-lowering drugs may soon be recommended by your physician as more is learned about their antistress benefits and their role in immune enhancement is more completely explored. In the meantime, you have another powerful reason for including vitamin C in your daily supplement program.

INFECTIOUS DISEASE CAN BE PSYCHOSOMATIC

Folk wisdom has always recognized that people with certain kinds of personalities get sick more often than others. In the twentieth century, it came to be recognized that certain diseases, such as ulcers, colitis, hyperthyroidism, rheumatoid arthritis, high blood pressure, asthma, and regional enteritis, tend to be associated with specific psychological problems. Unfortunately this created a false distinction between diseases that were considered psychosomatic and those that were thought to have a physical or organic cause.

Modern laboratory research is now beginning to confirm what our ancestors recognized from common sense observation — that psychological factors play a key role in a very wide range of diseases, and that the immune system is a critical mediator in the process.

Infectious diseases: the role of stress. Even though the concept of psychosomatic disease is well established, you may find it hard to accept that *infectious* disease can have a psychological element. If a disease is associated with a specific pathogen — as, for example, strep throat is associated with streptococcus — it seems reasonable to consider the streptococcus the cause of the disease. Yet a micro-organism alone may not be enough to produce illness. Many factors may affect your susceptibility — such as immunity from prior exposure to the pathogen, genetic influences, nutritional status, or the presence of another disease.

Psychological factors are most important in infectious diseases when there is a delicate balance between the host and the pathogen, and it takes another influence to tip the scales — that is, to determine whether the host eliminates the micro-organism, or becomes a carrier, or gets sick. Dosage of the pathogen is also important. If the disease-causing organism is present in very high concentration, the role of psychological factors is probably minimal, while a very low dosage of pathogen may not be enough to cause illness in any case (Plaut and Friedman 1981).

Because infectious diseases are often overlooked in the study of psychosomatic illness, only a few studies exist that show that the mind can influence your susceptibility to infectious disease.

One such study followed some cadets at West Point to see how psychological factors influenced their susceptibility to infectious mononucleosis. A group of cadets were selected at the beginning of the study who were all free of the antibody for the *Epstein-Barr virus,* which causes the disease — meaning that they had not previously been infected with the virus. During their stay at the academy, some of the young men developed the Epstein-Barr virus antibody; but only some of these actually developed mononucleosis. The others remained symptom free, indicating that they had better resistance. The cadets who became sick with infectious mononucleosis were generally found to have experienced greater academic pressure and to have shown poorer academic performance than the resistant group of cadets (Plaut and Friedman 1981).

In another group of students studied, it was found that failure, social isolation, or unresolved role crisis was often associated with respiratory infections. The more serious the sickness, the more likely it was that stressful situations had occurred during the preceding year (Palmblad 1981).

One tool used to relate psychological factors to the incidence of disease is a score of life change stress developed by Thomas Holmes and Richard Rahe of the University of Washington School of Medicine. A list of forty-two significant life events are assigned weighted scores according to their degree of stressfulness. These include both positive and negative experiences, since both can produce stress. Some examples of life change events, with their life stress scores, are: death of spouse (100), divorce (73), marriage (50), fired from job (47), retirement (45), change in residence (20), and vacation (13) (Holmes and Rahe 1967). In the typical study, a subject is asked to indicate which of these events has occurred during a given period of time, usually six to twenty-four months prior to testing. Generally it is found that the higher the life change score, the greater the likelihood that the person has suffered serious illness — including some infectious diseases — during the period under study.

The epidemiological studies we have described so far relate stress to the incidence of disease, but they ignore the hypothesized missing link — changes in the immune system that are brought about by stressful situations. Only a handful of studies have measured the impact of stressful events on specific immune functions. Such clinical studies typically involve following a group of people for a period of time, during which time changes in measures of their immune defenses are compared to changes in psychosocial factors.

Bereavement has very frequently been observed to have a damaging effect on health. In one of the first studies of its kind, a group of recently widowed women were tested for their immune responses at intervals following the death of their spouse. It was found that the T lymphocyte response to test cells (mitogens) was reduced approximately eight weeks following bereavement, as compared with testing shortly after bereavement (Palmblad 1981).

In another study, hypersensitivity reactions to immunization were found to occur more frequently in subjects who were rated as "vulnerable" according to a personality scale (Palmblad 1981).

Our Skylab astronauts are tested extensively to determine their reactions to their experience in space and to the stress of re-entry. During the first three days after splashdown, which presumably would be a very stressful event, T cell responses of the astronauts were found to be reduced (Palmblad 1981).

Sleep deprivation can also be a very stressful experience. A group of twelve healthy male students who were kept awake for forty-eight hours experienced a depression in cell-mediated immunity (Palmblad et al. 1979a, 1979b). A few days after the sleep deprivation period, cell function returned to normal and even appeared to be enhanced in some cases. This *rebound phenomenon* can sometimes work to our advantage in protecting us against disease, and it also helps to explain why some stress, properly handled, can be beneficial.

Animal studies. Laboratory-induced stress has frequently been shown to act as an immunosuppressant in animals. Such experiments have shown links between artificially induced stress and decreased resistance to viral infections as well as implanted tumors (Rogers et al. 1979). Induced stress in animals has been shown to depress B and T cell response, white cell toxicity, response to antigen, skin graft rejection, and delayed hypersensitivity reaction. In a series of graded stresses, the lymphocyte response was depressed in a correspondingly graded fashion (Keller et al. 1981).

One series of animal experiments showed that the immune response can actually be conditioned, in the same way that the famous Russian physiologist Pavlov conditioned dogs to salivate. In his pioneering work on classical conditioning, Pavlov observed that dogs salivated when they were presented with food. He then rang a bell just before the dogs were given their food, and after several repetitions of this procedure he observed that ringing the bell alone elicited salivation — a so-called conditioned response.

In a similar manner, researchers have been able to use classical conditioning to produce a suppression of the immune response. They gave mice a saccharin solution to drink at the same time that they injected the mice with cyclophosphamide, a drug that produces stomachache and that also happens to be an immuno-suppressant. After several repetitions, they found that the saccharin solution alone was enough to reduce the mice's immune response (Ader and Cohen 1981). (The researchers actually stumbled upon this finding in the course of conditioning the mice to have an aversion to saccharin, which they usually like. When the cyclophosphamide was stopped, the mice rapidly resumed drinking the saccharin, but some of them died. It was then that the investigators realized that cyclophosphamide was also an immunosuppressant and that drinking the saccharin was producing a conditioned immune suppression.)

This provocative study, and others that have repeated its findings, seem to have many potential implications for modifying immune responses in humans. If the immune response can be magnified through conditioning, as well as suppressed, it should be possible to enlist conditioning to enhance the effects of drugs (and placebos) and other forms of treatment.

How timing affects the immune response. In animal studies, the effect of stress on disease susceptibility varies, depending on when stress occurs in relation to exposure to a pathogen. There are three possibilities: stress may *precede* exposure to the pathogen; stress and pathogen exposure may occur at the *same time;* or stress may occur *after* pathogen exposure. When stress precedes the pathogen, there is sometimes increased resistance to the pathogen, while in the other two situations, resistance is always decreased (Palmblad 1981). While stress does suppress the immune response, that suppression may be for only a short period of time (if the stress is not chronic), and then the immune response comes back even more forcefully.

This rebound phenomenon was also observed in the sleep deprivation studies described earlier, indicating that it holds true for humans as well as for laboratory animals. The ability of the immune system to rebound may help to explain why some people actually thrive, mentally and physically, in a stressful environment where they are offered repeated opportunities to deal effectively with challenges.

STRESS MANAGEMENT

Of all the ways to avoid the harmful effects of stress on your immune functioning, by far the most effective is to learn to manage stress properly. It is easy to recognize the dangers of excess stress, but sometimes you may feel you are unable to prevent it. We will now discuss a few simple approaches to stress management that can help you to gain better control over your stress level, your immunity, and, therefore, your overall health.

Manage stress, don't avoid it. First, remember that stress is not necessarily a bad thing; in fact, according to Hans Selye, the "father of stress research," stress can be the spice of life. Meeting daily challenges successfully may actually produce a pleasant sensation that Selye calls "eustress." On the other hand, it is the "distress" of nonadaptation that is harmful to our health. Stress is a natural and potentially stimulating part of life; rather than seeking to avoid it altogether, we must develop ways of coping with it effectively.

You can do a great deal to control the stress induced by major events by ordering your life in a way that keeps too many significant life changes from happening all at the same time. If you are planning to get married, that is not a good time to change your job or move. After a divorce, you can try to maintain stability in other areas of your life by keeping your old eating and sleeping habits, pursuing your hobbies and special interests, and avoiding confrontations with your boss. Such stress management techniques, when events can be anticipated and planned for, can help to reduce the toll that life changes can take on your mental and physical well-being.

Of course, some events can't be scheduled in advance, and even in the absence of major life changes, we are exposed every day to stress-producing stimuli. In order to cope with the daily barrage of stressors, one key word to remember is *awareness*. Learn to recognize your own personal stress signals: racing heartbeat, clenching of the jaw, knotted stomach, tense muscles, racing thoughts —

whatever the sign of stress, stop right where you are and take a few minutes' time out. Breathe deeply ten times, or take a short walk. Learn to recognize what situations trigger this stress response and ask yourself how you can arrange your day to avoid such situations; or learn to redefine the situation so that it is no longer an annoyance.

Caffeine-containing drinks, including coffee, black tea, and colas, can contribute to stress if you drink too many. Try cutting down on caffeine drinks and switching to juices and herb teas. You may be surprised at the difference it makes in your stress level.

Relaxation techniques. Probably the most effective strategy for preventing the harmful effects of chronic stress is to learn how to relax. By systematically practicing relaxation techniques, you will enable your body to rebound from abnormal states of arousal and greatly increase your potential for good health. For optimal results, you should make a regular practice of fifteen or twenty minutes of deep, uninterrupted relaxation in a quiet place, every day.

There are many different techniques that can be practiced to achieve a profound state of relaxation, including meditation, deep breathing, visualization, progressive relaxation, autogenic training, biofeedback, or hypnotically induced relaxation, among others. You can find many books that explain such techniques in detail; or you may want to take a class that will introduce you to one of the more complex techniques.

Once you have mastered one of these relaxation techniques, you will find it even easier to recognize the signs of internal stress, and now you will have a tool to counteract it. It is impossible to exist in two contradictory states at the same time; you can not be distressed and relaxed simultaneously, and so if you manage to relax, the stress response will be alleviated.

Now that we have seen how stress can compromise immunity, and what you can do to reduce its harmful effects, let's take a look at the role of the mind in causing — and curing — some of the most troublesome diseases of the twentieth century.

CANCER: PSYCHOLOGICAL FACTORS

A cancer case history. John B. was a brilliant scientist working for a prestigious research firm. An overachiever all his life, John realized as he approached fifty that he hadn't gotten the recognition he had hoped for. He also regretted having given up a university teaching post to take the higher-paid research job. When he was put in charge of a major new project as a reward for his past breakthroughs, John was very unhappy at having to leave his old team; but he was unable to express these feelings to his employers.

Meanwhile, John's son went off to college. John and his son had shared a keen interest in sports; now John gave up attending sports events altogether. With their son gone, John and his wife were thrown together more and had increasing problems in communicating and in defining common interests.

At the age of fifty, John was diagnosed as having cancer of the pancreas, with a life expectancy of six to nine months (Simonton, Matthews-Simonton, and Creighton 1978).

Not everyone subjected to such a series of losses would respond, as John did, by developing cancer. In psychotherapy, John realized that part of his problem was that he placed everyone else's needs above his own. Working with his therapist, he learned to undo some of the damaging beliefs that kept him "trapped" in a disease-generating emotional state. Thus, it was his inability to cope with his losses, rather than the losses themselves, that probably weakened his defenses against cancer.

Is there a cancer-prone personality? As far back as the second century A.D., the Greek physician Galen observed that depressed women were more prone to cancer than cheerful women. Since then the medical literature has repeatedly reported that cancer appears to be associated with depression, anxiety, disappointment, and other similar emotions.

In the twentieth century, while medical interest in psychological determinants of disease has been on the wane, clinical psychologists have taken up the question and developed personality profiles of cancer patients. One such profile, developed by psychologist Lawrence LeShan (1977), finds that the lives of many cancer patients have the following points in common:

- marked by feelings of isolation, neglect, and despair as a youth, and having difficult interpersonal relationships
- in early adulthood, a consuming interest in either a strong and meaningful relationship or a satisfying vocation, which became the center of the person's life

- the loss of this relationship or role, resulting in despair and reactivating the painful feelings of childhood once again
- a characteristic "bottling up" of despair; while cancer patients are often described by other people as kind, sweet, and benign, this sweetness is really a mask they wear to conceal their feelings of anger, hurt, and hostility.

The stress of life changes alone does not induce the development of cancer. There must also be an underlying personality structure that handles such life changes in an unhealthy way. Feelings of loneliness and hopelessness, of being helpless or trapped, often characterize people who develop this dread disease.

Animal experiments also suggest that a sense of helplessness plays a role in cancer causation. In such experiments, rats were injected with cancer cells and then divided into different groups. Some were exposed to electric shock that they could escape, while a second group were unable to escape the shock. A control group received no shock at all. The rats who were exposed to the escapable shock were able to reject the implanted cancer cells significantly more effectively than the rats who had no way of escaping. That is, the cancer grew fastest and led to the earliest deaths among the animals who had no means of coping with their stress. The rats who received the same amount of shock but were able to act to evade it had about the same rate of tumor growth as the control group who received no shocks at all (Vistainer et al. 1982).

Stress, immunity, and cancer. According to medical thinking, cancer begins with a critical mutation in the cells. Such a mutation might be produced by any number of factors, including radiation, chemicals, viruses, hormones, physical irritants, or even aging alone. Such a change in cells is not enough in itself to produce cancer. In fact, such potentially cancerous cells are probably being produced in all our bodies from time to time, but our immune systems are usually able to eliminate them.

The immune system has many weapons against tumors, including B and T cells, natural killer cells, and macrophages. Noncellular weapons against cancer include antibodies, interferons, and *complement*. Complement is another important element of immune system functioning. The term describes a complex series of activities of enzymatic serum protein which influence the antigen-antibody reaction. When antibody attaches to an antigen, the antibody may undergo physicochemical changes that attract an enzyme system in the area. This enzyme system is made up of several different complement components, which participate in different immune functions. Through a series of combinations and alterations, complement activity thus results, for example, in more effective phagocytosis, virus neutralization, chemotaxis (chemical attraction), and cytolysis (cell splitting).

Many animal studies suggest that stress can suppress these immune system mechanisms, opening the way for cancer; but it is not always easy to extrapolate from animal studies to humans. Laboratory experiments generally expose the animals to much more potent cancer-causing influences (such as radiation or implanted tumors) than humans usually experience. Moreover, viruses account for a large proportion of spontaneous cancers in the rodents used in laboratories, while viruses are not now believed to be responsible for many human cancers.

Poor coping suppresses cancer-fighting cells. Studies of humans are now verifying that stress, and how well we cope with it, can have a direct effect on cancer-fighting components of the immune system.

Earlier in this chapter, we looked at some studies showing how stress influences specific immune functions in humans. Another such study (Locke et al. 1979) found that the activity of cancer-fighting natural killer cells can be influenced by psychological factors. Natural killer cell activity was measured in healthy human subjects and compared with life change stress scores and the incidence of psychiatric symptoms during the previous year. Significantly, life changes themselves did not necessarily correlate with suppression of NK cell activity; rather it was the *interaction* of life change stress and psychiatric symptoms that was the most important factor. Natural killer cell activity was highest among those with high levels of life change stress but few symptoms, and lowest among those with both high life change stress and many psychiatric symptoms. This shows that our *ability to cope* with the stress of life changes affects our natural killer cell activity — a key measure of cancer resistance (Fox 1981).

Healing cancer with the mind. Psychological factors not only influence the development of cancer, but they may also play a critical role in recovery. The outcome of cancer treatment can very often be influenced by the patient's beliefs and expectations about how effective the treatment is and how potent the body's natural defenses are.

This idea is being applied in clinical practice, using psychological processes to enhance the immune defenses of cancer patients. Typically patients are put in a state of deep relaxation and then asked to visualize their disease, the therapy they are receiving, and the white cells in their immune system; the therapy and the white cells are then visualized winning the battle against the disease. This combination of deep relaxation and positive visualization is believed to put the patients in touch with processes that are generally considered beyond their conscious control.

The unquestioned leaders in the use of these techniques in cancer therapy are Carl and Stephanie Simonton. The Simontons combined their respective backgrounds in radiation therapy and motivational psychology in an attempt to awaken the self-healing powers of their patients' minds and bodies. By encouraging patients to participate actively in their cancer treatment, the Simontons have been achieving remarkable results. As they reported in their ground-breaking book *Getting Well Again* (1978):

> We began studying a group of patients with malignancies deemed medically incurable. Expected survival time for the average patient with such a malignancy is twelve months.
>
> In the past four years, we have treated 159 patients with a diagnosis of medically incurable malignancy. Sixty-three of the patients are alive, with an average survival of 24.4 months since the diagnosis. . . . With the patients in our study who have died, their average survival time was 20.3 months. In other words, the patients in our study who are alive have lived, on the average, two times longer than patients who received medical treatment alone. Even those patients in the study who have died still lived one and one-half times longer than the control group.

We must emphasize that the Simonton approach does *not replace* conventional cancer therapy with a psychological approach. Rather it uses the visualization work as an adjunct to surgery, chemotherapy, radiation, and/or other medical approaches. Many patients enter cancer therapy with negative expectations, having heard that chemotherapy or radiation will make them sick. Similarly, many people consider a diagnosis of cancer as a virtual death sentence, even though a very high proportion of cancer patients are surviving today. The Simontons find that their relaxation and visualization techniques can help the patients to create more positive expectations about the outcome of their disease and the effectiveness of their therapy, and that these positive expectations help to bring about remissions and often complete recovery.

In the course of recovery, the patients eventually have to confront the stress-producing emotional problems that contributed to their illness in the first place; but bolstered by their new, positive expectations, they are generally able to make progress in this area also. And so, the Simontons report, many patients who manage to survive the challenge of a bout with cancer emerge from the experience more healthy than they were to begin with.

Obviously this sort of process could work equally well in helping patients recover from other kinds of illnesses and in improving the efficacy of drugs and other forms of treatment. Considering how fearful people are of cancer, the success of the Simontons' approach is powerful testimony to the tremendous potential of the mind to stimulate the body's healing powers.

AIDS patients have a highly increased risk of cancer because of their immune deficiency. We will see in Chapter 10 that Russ Jaffe, M.D., Ph.D., is able to work with eighteen AIDS patients to achieve remission for eighteen months, through a combination of immunity-boosting approaches bolstered by self-image enhancement therapy.

The message from such promising work is clear. If you, or someone you know, is diagnosed as having cancer, don't panic and think that your *only* objective is to get rid of the cancer. Cutting out a cancer does not resolve the underlying circumstances, which may include psychological or nutritional problems among others. If a plant begins to wilt or turn brown, you fertilize the soil; you shouldn't simply cut off the withered leaves. Fertilizing the soil of your body by providing proper nutrients is a very important step in cancer recovery. Looking at underlying psychological conflicts, and coming to terms with them, might be compared to cultivating and weeding in order to provide a healthier groundwork for returning to good health.

As many scientists/healers are learning, the process of recovering from cancer often entails confronting an underlying stressful situation. By recognizing cancer as a message from the body that something needs to be resolved, people can use the disease as an opportunity to make radical improvements in their mental and physical health.

AUTOIMMUNE DISEASES AND THE MIND

Barbara M. was seriously depressed. An athletic army officer in her mid-thirties, she was proud of her independence and constantly strove for perfection. The only woman active in major international sports-car racing, she had wrecked her Maserati and was not doing as well using a substitute car. When she sought help for her depression, her doctor immediately recognized her as a prime candidate for autoimmune disease. He then took her history and learned that she had had idiopathic thrombocytopenic purpura (a possible autoimmune disease) two years earlier. Her laboratory tests revealed that she had a high antinuclear antibody count* in her blood. Three months later, she came down with the autoimmune disease systemic lupus erythematosus (Solomon 1981a).

It is interesting that her doctor, when he first met Barbara M., immediately spotted her as a likely person to have an autoimmune disease. Her perfectionism, her athletic interests, and the depression that followed on her accident — as well as the fact that she was a woman — are traits she shared with many other sufferers from lupus, rheumatoid arthritis, and other autoimmune disorders.

Just as there seem to be certain personality traits that predispose people to cancer, so are some of the autoimmune diseases associated with specific personality variables, which in turn may influence the immune system.

In the case of cancer, we have said that overactive T suppressor cells may help allow cancer to develop. For autoimmune diseases, the situation appears to be just the opposite — inadequate T suppressor cell function. Even though T suppressor cells tend to slow down the immune response, a lack of these important regulatory cells is still an immune deficiency and may be a result of emotional distress, among other causes.

---

*A laboratory test that helps to detect autoimmune disease.

Personality and stress in rheumatoid arthritis. Of all the autoimmune diseases, rheumatoid arthritis (RA) has been studied most extensively to define an associated personality type. Over the years, a picture of the typical rheumatoid arthritic has emerged. According to Dr. George Solomon (1981a), who has studied the psychological component of autoimmune diseases extensively, "the arthritic process is not merely frequently, but always, the expression of a personality conflict." Arthritic patients tend to turn their anger inward, rather than openly express their feelings. Here is how Solomon describes the personality of RA patients:

> Rheumatoid arthritics were extremely dependent, felt inadequate, had difficulty coping with their environment and with other people, and were severely blocked in emotional expression. They frequently denied their dependency by overcompensating with an outward facade of independence, self-assurance, and self-control. Their attitude towards work and responsibility varied from an attempt to negate their dependence, both by accepting far more responsibility than they could handle and by overwork, to a manifestation of their dependency and inadequacy by avoidance of all responsibility and reliance upon others for guidance. They avoided closeness, were aware of strong unexpressible angry feelings, reacted oversensitively to the slightest criticism or rejection, and tended to court others' favor, allowing themselves to deal with their tensions defensively by varying degrees of overactivity.... The single most important precipitating factor was the loss of, or separation from, important key figures upon whom these patients depended for support. (Solomon 1981a)

To test the validity of this personality profile, Solomon and his coworkers set up a study comparing female RA patients with their chronologically closest sisters who did not have rheumatoid arthritis, to see if there were personality trends common to the arthritics but not shared by their nonarthritic sisters (Solomon 1981a). Thus the control group was as closely matched to the study group as possible, in terms of family background, sex, age, and other genetic and environmental influences.

The arthritic patients scored significantly higher on scales measuring "perfectionism, compliance and subservience, nervousness and restlessness, reserve and introversion, depression and sensitivity (to anger)" compared to their sisters. The arthritics described themselves with adjectives such as "nervous, tense, worried, struggling, depressed, moody, highly strung, and easily upset," whereas their nonarthritic sisters described themselves as "liking people, easy to get acquainted with, enjoying life in a generally unruffled manner." Whereas the RA patients were martyr-like and masochistic in their relationships with their husbands, their nonarthritic sisters were able to express anger at their spouses and children when they were provoked. Almost every RA patient in the Solomon study traced the development of her arthritis to an acute or chronic stress situation.

Children can develop RA also, although the role of personality and stress in their case has not been as well studied. In one survey, which compared eighty-eight children who had RA against a random pediatric population, it was found that among the arthritics there was a high incidence of youngsters whose parents had been divorced, separated, or widowed. Adoption had occurred three times more frequently among the RA children than among the comparison group. Fifty-one percent of these traumatic events occurred near the onset of the children's disease (Solomon 1981a).

Strong as the evidence for psychological factors in RA may be, we must remember the biology professor's edict, "Microbes *do* exist." Illness is not entirely psychosomatic in origin. We will follow up this discussion of rheumatoid arthritis in Chapter 11 by reporting on thirty years of research implicating *protozoa* in this crippling disease, and we will also review evidence that RA incidence may be related to levels of iron in the diet.

Other autoimmune diseases. There are also typical personality profiles for autoimmune diseases besides RA. *Ulcerative colitis* is often associated with antibodies that attack the colon, and so may be autoimmune in nature. Patients having this disease were described as having "obsessive-compulsive traits of neatness, indecision, conscientiousness, worrying, rigid morality, and conformity" and also had difficulty expressing hostility. *Systemic lupus erythematosus** often has its onset following an episode of stress, especially the loss of a significant relationship or fear of the loss of love.

---

*Please see Chapter 11 for details of this disease, alarmingly on the increase among young, vital women.

Lupus is also often associated with depression and with an unusual need for activity and independence (Solomon 1981a). Looking back once again at the case of Barbara M., the race car driver, you will see why she was likely to come down with an autoimmune disease.

Is schizophrenia an autoimmune disease? A number of immune system abnormalities have been found among people with serious psychiatric disorders, and particularly schizophrenia. It is possible that abnormal central nervous system function might be influencing the immune system; but on the other hand, perhaps abnormal immunological factors are producing the mental illness. Of particular interest is the fact that *antibrain antibodies* (which attack the brain) have been found in the blood of mental patients:

> A variety of immunologic abnormalities has been reported in conjunction with mental illness, particularly schizophrenia. These findings include abnormalities in levels of immunoglobulins; abnormal heterophile antibodies; the presence of autoantibodies to a variety of self components, including the presence of antibrain antibodies; deficient immune responsivity; and morphological and functional abnormalities of immunologically competent cells (Solomon 1981b).

Among the immunoglobulin abnormalities found in schizophrenics are elevated levels of IgA and IgM. Elevations of these two antibodies are also found in autoimmune diseases such as rheumatoid arthritis and lupus. Antinuclear antibodies were found to be elevated in mentally ill and mentally deficient hospitalized psychiatric patients and are also characteristic of lupus.

There may also be a strong genetic component that predisposes certain people toward having both immune problems and schizophrenia. One piece of evidence supporting such a genetic connection is the fact that abnormal white cells have been found with high frequency in schizophrenics and their family members (Solomon 1981b).

Why women? One of the great unsolved mysteries of the autoimmune diseases is why they affect women so much more frequently than men. According to one researcher, "the majority of patients suffering from various types of autoimmune diseases are female, and most of these diseases have peculiar age distributions which seem to be related to periods characterized by physiological endocrine alterations" (Ahlqvist 1981). Thus mid-life is a typical time for the appearance of many autoimmune diseases, just as it is a time of great hormonal change.

While hormonal changes relating to events such as menopause may certainly be a factor in these diseases, the psychological impact of such events may be an equally important factor. For example, it has been observed that rheumatoid arthritis and other autoimmune diseases often improve during pregnancy, even though progesterone (the hormone associated with pregnancy) and placental extracts have *not* been helpful in treating arthritis. After childbirth the symptoms sometimes get worse once again.

If psychological factors do play a part in autoimmune diseases, perhaps the role conflicts inherent in the position of women in today's society are responsible. This would help to explain why these diseases are so much more common in women. For example, women have traditionally been expected not to express anger. As we have mentioned, holding back anger appears to be a common trait among people with rheumatoid arthritis, and perhaps other autoimmune diseases as well. Similarly, no matter how strongly a woman may feel about childbearing or not having children, she is still likely to feel some conflict about the decision which may be aggravated or resolved by such events as pregnancy or menopause.

Psychotherapy may help autoimmune diseases. Fortunately the connection between immune problems and psychological disturbances can work in either direction. Not only can emotional factors contribute to the development of autoimmune diseases, but they can also provide clues to their treatment. The Persian physician Razi recognized this principle more than one thousand years ago, when he used psychotherapy to treat a patient with rheumatoid arthritis. Razi felt that the patient's arthritic condition was connected to his inability to experience and express aggression.

If people who develop rheumatoid arthritis tend to hold back their anger, then relatively harmless situations may be the cause of intolerable stress for them, leading to abnormalities in immune functions. Psychotherapy may be able to aid these people in expressing their anger, thus helping them to recover or preventing flare-ups in their disease.

A similar therapeutic process may be helpful in other autoimmune diseases. One physician reported that a patient whose lupus had progressed to the point of kidney damage was able to achieve a remission by "dumping" on her father her long-concealed and unexpressed hostility (Solomon 1981a).

Many people with autoimmune diseases feel frustration and anger about the public's lack of understanding of their illness. Sufferers from many autoimmune diseases seem to derive significant benefit from support groups in which they are allowed to share their concerns and explore their conflicts in a safe and understanding environment.

PSYCHOSOMATIC HEALTH

For some reason, people seem to find it easier to accept that the mind can make us sick than that it can help us get well. Yet two people with the same sort of disease and the same treatment will often have quite different outcomes, one dying or becoming permanently disabled and the other recovering completely. The only thing that seems to distinguish them is something we vaguely define as their "will to live."

Until recently the notion of psychosomatic healing was largely dismissed as some sort of superstition. Now we have discovered, through the use of psychological tools such as biofeedback, that we are capable of exerting conscious control over many processes — such as pulse rate, blood pressure, and body temperature — that previously were thought to be involuntary. Similarly, it used to be felt that the mind/body connection in disease must be unconscious in nature, and therefore there was not much we could do about it even if it did exist. Now, as we have seen, some of the most promising work in stimulating immune function is being done not with drugs but with psychotherapy, helping patients with immune disorders to recover from sometimes life-threatening illnesses.

Getting help. If stress and psychological conflict can help to *cause* disease, then clearly these problems need to be resolved as part of your response to an illness. You may understand intellectually that holding back your true feelings, or driving yourself from one stressful situation to another, is "eating away" at you;

but if you don't do something to change your response to stress, your ulcer or asthma or arthritis or cancer is not likely to go away. Counseling — of many different sorts — can be an effective adjunct to medical treatment. Support groups exist for people with most of the principal immune diseases of adulthood, from lupus to AIDS to cancer. You can locate such groups through the associations supporting research and public education about these diseases, such as the Arthritis Foundation, the American Cancer Society, or the Lupus Foundation of America.

Many people are reluctant to seek psychological counseling because they think it would be an admission that they are mentally ill. Now that you understand how intimately your mind is connected to your immune functioning, you can see that counseling can be simply another tool for improving your immunity.

HOW THE BRAIN REGULATES IMMUNITY

It may surprise you that the role of the brain is a relatively new "discovery" in the unfolding mystery of immunity. For a long time, scientists thought that the immune system operated entirely on its own, responding directly to the threats of internal or external antigens.

Studies of immune functions are often conducted outside the body, observing the interaction of cells under a microscope. Such a wide range of immune processes occur under these isolated, artificial conditions that some researchers have felt there is no need to bring the brain into the picture. However, researchers in the new field of psychoneuroimmunology are uncovering the facts about the many ways that the nervous system can enhance, regulate, or suppress the immune response. These findings offer some valuable clues about what we can do to improve our immunity.

The neurotransmitters. Among the brain's most important tools in regulating immunity are the *neurotransmitters*, chemical messengers that stimulate nervous system mechanisms throughout the body.

Proper functioning of the nervous system depends on the rapid transmission of nerve impulses from one nerve cell to the next. The neurotransmitters, secreted at the nerve endings, are responsible for transmitting signals between nerve cells.

While there are several different neurotransmitters, three main kinds have an influence on the immune system. *Acetylcholine* is a neurotransmitter that stimulates nervous system function. A deficiency of brain acetylcholine has been found in the debilitating, memory-destroying Alzheimer's disease. *Serotonin* is an inhibitory neurotransmitter involved in cognitive functions, mental illness, and sleep cycles. The psychedelic drug LSD has a strikingly similar chemical structure to serotonin. *Dopamine* and the related *norepinephrine* (a form of adrenalin present in the nervous system), a third class of neurotransmitters, are known as *catecholamines*. Dopamine deficiency is a characteristic of Parkinson's disease, which is marked by muscular tremor. Because many antipsychotic drugs block dopamine transmission from one neuron to another, these drugs give rise to Parkinson's-like side effects.

Acetylcholine has been shown, at least indirectly, to have an influence on the immune system. Thymus tissue contains receptors for acetylcholine, and the neurotransmitter also stimulates a nucleic acid product that activates B and T cells. Acetylcholine also seems to stimulate stem cells in the bone marrow, enhancing the production of B and T cells. On the whole, stimulation of acetylcholine production seems to increase B cell and T cell response (Hall and Goldstein 1981).

There is much stronger evidence for the role of serotonin, which seems to have an inhibitory influence over immune functions. There appears to be an inverse relation between brain serotonin levels and antibody production. Injection of the immediate precursor of serotonin decreases antibody response, while decreased brain serotonin results in increased immunity (Hall and Goldstein 1981). It seems paradoxical that serotonin should be an immunosuppressant, since its calmative effects on the nervous system are so beneficial overall. Perhaps as research reveals more about this neurotransmitter's effect on the nervous system, this mystery will be unraveled.

Dopamine appears to have an overall stimulant effect on various immune functions, based on evidence from diseases that affect the dopamine pathways, such as Parkinson's disease. Parkinson's patients (who have a dopamine deficiency) are observed to have reductions in T cells and in T cell response. In contrast, B cell response may be increased by dopamine shortage. When given to young mice, L-dopa (which increases dopamine levels), the drug used to treat Parkinson's disease, produced a youthful appearance and a significantly prolonged life span — presumably because of its immune-enhancing effects (Hall and Goldstein 1981).

Table 3 summarizes the *known* effects of the neurotransmitters on immune functions.

TABLE 3

How Neurotransmitters Affect the Immune System

Neurotransmitter	B cell response	T cell response	Macrophages	Stem cells in bone marrow
Elevated serotonin	Decrease	No data	No data	No data
Elevated dopamine	Decrease	Increase	Increase	Increase
Elevated acetylcholine	Increase	Increase	No data	Increase

Source: Hall and Goldstein, 1981

Using amino acids to boost neurotransmitters. Many people today are using amino acids, the building blocks that make up proteins, to affect brain function. You can take amino acids to become more alert or to help you sleep, to alter your mood or to control your appetite. The rationale behind taking extra amino acids is that they are required to boost the levels of neurotransmitters in the nervous system.

This means that *your diet has a direct effect on the balance of neurotransmitters in your brain.* Richard Wurtman, M.D., a neuroendocrinologist at the Massachusetts Institute of Technology in Cambridge and one of the pioneers in investigating the influence of nutrients on brain function, expressed his amazement at the neurotransmitters' susceptibility to outside manipulation:

It remains peculiar to me that the brain should have evolved in such a way that it is subject to having its function and chemistry depend on whether you had lunch, and what you ate. I would not have designed the brain that way myself. (Quoted in Weisburd 1984)

Of the neurotransmitters we have discussed, three are known to be subject to dietary control. The amino acid precursor for serotonin is *tryptophan;* the precursor for norepinephrine (a derivative of dopamine) is the amino acid *tyrosine;* and that for acetylcholine is the amino acid *choline.* The amount of each of these neurotransmitters in the brain is influenced by how much of its respective amino acid precursor is present.

How do we get these amino acids into the brain? In the case of acetylcholine, the process is straightforward. An increase in blood choline levels rapidly leads to an increase in brain choline concentration, and acetylcholine production is stimulated. Choline is normally present in the diet in the fatty acid *lecithin,* which occurs, for example, in eggs and fish. Thus eating lecithin increases blood and brain choline levels, stimulating the production of acetylcholine.

The mechanism for increasing brain serotonin is more complicated. Eating high-protein food will actually have the net effect of *reducing* the amount of the amino acid tryptophan, the serotonin precursor, in the brain. This is because a complex system is required to transport tryptophan into the brain across the blood-brain barrier (capillary walls and other membranes that separate the blood from the interior of the central nervous system organs). When pure tryptophan is taken, brain tryptophan and serotonin levels rapidly rise, as long as no other proteins are ingested; but if other animal proteins are consumed, the competing amino acids prevent much of the tryptophan from getting past the blood-brain barrier. The relative concentration of tryptophan is thus reduced, and serotonin production is not stimulated.

Paradoxically, the meal that is most likely to enhance brain tryptophan and serotonin concentration is one containing carbohydrate and no proteins. Carbohydrate induces the production of insulin, which reduces the levels of competing amino acids in the blood stream, but does not affect tryptophan levels, leaving the tryptophan free to enter the brain. Of course taking a tryptophan supplement along with a high-carbohydrate, low-protein meal will also increase brain serotonin.

Norepinephrine appears to be stimulated by the presence of its amino acid precursor, tyrosine. As with tryptophan, combining tyrosine with carbohydrates may enhance the amino acid's ability to induce norepinephrine production.

Using amino acids for health problems. The use of amino acids to stimulate neurotransmitter production already has many clinical applications. (See Appendix 2.) For example, tryptophan, by increasing serotonin levels, can be helpful in controlling carbohydrate cravings, and thus shows promise in helping to correct eating disorders. Tryptophan is useful for inducing sleep and, in combination with antidepressant drugs, in improving mood in depressed patients. It is helpful as a pain killer, and perhaps in stimulating growth hormone secretion.

Tyrosine is believed to work as an antidepressant by stimulating the production of norepinephrine. It is credited with increasing mental alertness, improving memory, and creating a positive, immunity-enhancing mood. Tyrosine also produces a dramatic reduction in the blood pressure of hypertensive rats. This unexpected finding is likely to stimulate even greater interest in this amino acid in the future.

The use of choline, often in combination with lecithin, to stimulate acetylcholine production has shown promising results in the treatment of senile dementia and Alzheimer's disease, with an improvement in cognitive function and in patients' ability to take care of themselves. Many of the diseases of aging have been linked to faulty acetylcholine transmission, and Alzheimer's disease specifically is characterized by the loss of nerve cells that produce acetylcholine.

Strategies for using amino acids as supplements. Getting the greatest benefit from amino acids depends on balancing them properly with other nutrients. For example, reducing dietary protein generally improves the efficacy of amino acids taken as drugs or supplements. Carbohydrates, in combination with tryptophan and possibly also with tyrosine, seem to maximize the amino acid's effect in treating diseases.

Certain vitamins also are essential to proper utilization of amino acids to produce neurotransmitters. Tryptophan, when taken along with vitamins B_3 and B_6, seems to be even more effective in controlling psychiatric symptoms. Tryptophan combined with vitamin B_3 makes it possible to reduce the dosage of the antidepressive drug imipramine (Levine 1980).

Obviously, using amino acids properly is a very complex matter. To avoid any possible undesirable effects (such as overstimulation) and save yourself unnecessary expense, be sure to consult with a qualified nutritionist to determine your individual needs before experimenting with these potentially powerful nutrients.

Looking again at the Master Sheet of mind/body connections (on the next page), we see how a program of attitudinal modification will produce an improved score for psychoneuroimmunological health. A person, either adult or child, who scores highly on this portion of the Im.Q. test will more than likely be in psychological harmony. This is not to say that such a person will not experience pain, disappointment, frustration, anger, hostility, or other "negative" emotions. But they will know how to deal with such feelings before they simmer beneath the surface and bring about biochemical changes on a cellular-immunological level.

Religion, like psychology, is an attempt to bring peace to the individual (when properly applied). But in recent years, we have learned that talk, ritual, even tranquilizers can go only so far to keep a person in relative balance. To go beyond medicating ourselves into a state of momentary peace, to achieve true harmony, we must incorporate nutrition and exercise — the topics of our next three chapters.

Together, mind, diet, and physical movement will unify our forces of immunity.

THE MASTER SHEET

(Mind/Body Connections)

Have not had a major illness in years. *10 pts.*	Have never suffered from allergies. *9 pts.*	Do not feel like an "outsider." *8 pts.*
Am generally confident. *7 pts.*	Cuts heal rapidly. *6 pts.*	Reasonably satisfied with career, income, or school. *5 pts.*
Am not more than 10 lbs. over ideal weight. *4 pts.*	Have a circle of close friends. *3 pts.*	Readily get rid of rage, anger, hostility, and aggression. *2 pts.*

Your score _____

Maximum score this block _____ 54 _____

∘ 5 ∘

Nutrition Against Immunity

NUTRITIONAL ADVICE for enhancing immunity must begin with some elimination procedures. Before telling you about *protective* foods (in the next chapter), I would like to talk about *deficit* foods, those that do not add but subtract from our Immunity Quotient.

You can get your mind in order, run a few miles a day, keep your sexuality under control, and otherwise maintain yourself, but all of this can be upset by eating foods that are contaminated or inherently harmful, which puts them in the deficit column of nutritional/immunological health.

Red meat, refined flour, white sugar, and food additives have been "beaten to death" in the popular health literature since Robert Rodale, Adelle Davis, and other pioneer health teachers drummed into their readers the very real dangers of using these foods to excess.

Most enlightened readers take vitamins on a regular basis and try (as far as possible) to substitute pure foods, fruits, vegetables, fish, and whole grains for the previous diet of meat and potatoes.

Besides its other dangers, we now know that a diet of refined and processed foods, or one high in fats, is dangerous to your immune functioning. In this chapter, we will show which specific foods and substances depress immunity and how to avoid them. The next chapter clearly details the compensatory foods and nutrients that stimulate immunity.

We want to begin with a new artificial sweetener because of its falsely lauded safety and the enormous amount of it that is being used. Sugar already steals from our nutritional/immunological balance sheet by taking the place of protective foods. While we do not have direct evidence that this artificial sweetener suppresses immunity, we do know that each gram that goes into your body eliminates one gram of immune-enhancing nutrients that you would otherwise take.

By mid-1985, one key ingredient of aspartame, the amino acid phenylalanine, was implicated as causing brain damage in developing fetuses. Dr. Louis Elsas, director of medical genetics at Emory University in Atlanta, and Dr. Reuben Matalon, professor of pediatrics and genetics at the University of Illinois Medical School, extensively studied both aspartame and phenylalanine. They concluded that one woman in fifty is very sensitive to large doses of the amino acid and if those women consume this artificial sweetener during pregnancy, "it may cause birth defects." In addition to being a threat to pregnant women, the sweetener may also be dangerous for infants, these researchers concluded. Another researcher, Dr. Keith Connors of D.C. Children's Hospital reported of a case where a five-year-old child became emotionally uncontrollable after drinking sodas that contained aspartame. The patient "reportedly ran full force into the wall, knocking himself to the floor, crying, and repeating the performance until he was restrained."

IS ASPARTAME (EQUAL, NUTRASWEET) SAFE FOR ADULTS?

The most recent entry in the parade of low-calorie artificial sweeteners, aspartame was approved for consumer use in 1981. This protein-based product, marketed under the brand names Equal and NutraSweet, is about two hundred times sweeter than white sugar, or sucrose, and so provides fewer calories for equivalent sweetening power. Its predecessors, such as cyclamate and saccharin, have been implicated as known or possible *carcinogens* — cancer-causing substances — but aspartame received a clean bill of health from the FDA. However, it is generally used to sweeten cold foods, since it tends to lose its sweetness when heated.* Even worse, one of the products aspartame breaks down into in the digestive tract, methanol, is toxic. What happens after aspartame breaks down into its constituents — the amino acids aspartic acid and phenylalanine — is that methanol (wood alcohol) is formed! Many foods in nature contain methanol, including drinking alcohol; but most sources of methanol in nature are accompanied by ethanol, and it turns out that ethanol is a specific antidote for methanol. It was once common practice in medical circles to treat a child who had drunk some methanol by pumping his stomach quickly and then giving him plenty of a high grade of ethanol — keeping him drunk for a few days. Apparently the same enzyme that breaks up ethanol into acetaldehyde also breaks up methanol into formaldehyde. Now, acetaldehyde is mildly toxic, but the body can metabolize it slowly. In high amounts, this is what produces a hangover. The enzyme that does this far prefers ethanol to methanol; so if you can bind up all this enzyme with ethanol, then the methanol is not metabolized. If the methanol simply remained methanol in the body, it would be harmless, since it would be excreted. But instead, it metabolizes into formaldehyde. To prevent methanol from doing that, you should drink some ethanol. You might mix your alcoholic drinks with Tab, but we wouldn't advise drinking Tab without mixing it with alcohol!

HEAVY METALS REDUCE IMMUNITY

Our food, water, and air have steadily become contaminated with the heavy metals lead, cadmium, and mercury. In animal studies, these metals suppress all aspects of immune functioning, reducing cell-mediated and humoral immunity, depressing phagocyte responses, and increasing susceptibility to infection (Gordon 1983). Even at low levels not generally considered toxic, these contaminants can produce serious damage, especially to the nervous system. Growing children are particularly endangered by such low-level heavy metal exposure (Weiner 1981).

---

*Unfortunately, a modified form of aspartame has now been introduced in drinks that are heated. For example, it is being used as a substitute for sugar in "gourmet" coffee mixes. The breakdown products formed by heating aspartame are of unknown safety.

A major source of cadmium is cigarette smoke, which creates an increased risk of vascular disease not only for smokers but also for nonsmokers who inhale the fumes (Gordon 1983). Organic fertilizers made from sewage sludge often lead to dangerous cadmium levels in produce. Elevated cadmium levels have been shown to impair host resistance, antibody response, B and T cell response, and phagocyte response (Beisel 1982) and to depress bone marrow function (Weiner 1981).

Most of us know about lead and mercury, the origins of these toxic metals, and how to avoid them. Cadmium is less well understood. This is unfortunate because this toxic metal is appearing through all levels of society at increasingly alarming rates.

Cadmium is entering our bodies from food, air, and water. This metal is a by-product of heavy industry. Factory workers exposed to cadmium oxide dust often develop emphysema or, with high-level exposures, an acute "or even fatal pneumonia" (NAS 1973).

In our home, this metal enters our body through many sources. Cadmium-plated trays and vessels, or soft water that remains in contact with galvanized or black polyethylene pipes, have been isolated as sources of this toxin. Hypertension has been correlated with this metal in certain studies, but not definitively.

If you suspect your exposure to this metal has been high, you may want to have your serum zinc level analyzed. The reason is that cadmium competes with zinc, and signs of zinc deficiency may indicate high cadmium levels. By taking extra zinc in a vitamin/mineral supplement, for example, you will also be compensating for any excess of this toxic waste product that you may have ingested.

Most people today have a lead level five hundred times higher than our ancestors did (Gordon 1983), owing to automobile exhaust and other air pollution, lead-containing paints, and the presence of lead in food and water. Rural dwellers have been found to have the lowest lead levels on hair analysis, with urban groups higher, and the highest being people who live close to lead smelters. Excess lead has been found to impair host resistance and possibly antibody response and to inhibit B and T cell proliferation and reticuloendothelial response* (Beisel 1982). Brain dam-

---

*See Table 7 in Chapter 6 for a description of this and other technical terms.

age, neuritis, and kidney cancer are among the harmful conse-quences of lead toxicity (James 1982).

Mercury is a frequent contaminant of fish and shellfish. An ex-cess of this metal inhibits host resistance and antibody response, causes lymphoid tissue changes, and may bring about an autoim-mune attack on the kidney (Beisel 1982). The contamination of our food supply with mercury is a growing, not a diminishing, problem. But, rather than scare ourselves away from a major source of protective nutrients — including first-rate protein, namely fish — we can rest easy. Man-created mercury pollution of freshwater rivers and lakes will increase the mercury levels in *freshwater* fish. However, fish from the open oceans are generally safe. Museum specimens of tuna caught between seventy and one hundred years ago were found to contain the same range of mer-cury levels as those found in five more recently caught tuna. So, eat your ocean fish, and avoid the questionable shellfish from in-land waters as well as fish from lakes and rivers with marginal ecological health.

As with other heavy metals, avoiding contaminated foods and waters is a first step in detoxifying, or keeping your body load to a minimal level. But here as in other areas, political activism will be required to make our air, waters, and lands safe for human and animal life — now and in the future.

Your fillings may be poisoning you! Mercury is also a compo-nent of the amalgam used in dental fillings. Although dental amalgam has generally been considered safe, many people are known to have allergic reactions to it, usually in the form of skin rashes. Of even greater concern is the possibility of immune sup-pression and other toxic effects from mercury slowly transferring out of fillings into your cells. One dentist experimentally removed amalgam fillings from three patients and observed an *increase* in the proportion of T cells. When the amalgam was restored, the T cell percentages dropped again. This study suggests that amalgam fillings chronically depress these vital fighting cells in the immune system (Eggleston 1984). (Remember, reduced T cell percentages can increase the risk of cancer, infectious disease, and autoim-mune diseases.)

Alloys of nickel, a known carcinogen, are also used in dental work. In the study reported above, nickel also was found to have an adverse effect on T cell percentages.

Progressive dentists now strongly suspect that amalgam and nickel alloys should not be used in the mouth, and some people are having their fillings removed and replaced with potentially less toxic plastic compounds.

Hair analysis. As we have seen, heavy metal exposure is virtually inescapable today. Hair analysis is proving to be a useful and sensitive tool for identifying dangerous levels of these toxic substances. Hair analysis was sometimes unreliable in the past, owing to faulty techniques and limitations in the technology. Today standardized procedures for collection, preparation, and testing of hair samples have made hair analysis a reliable indicator of levels of harmful minerals (Gordon 1983). Another reliable indicator of mercury levels in our body can be had through serum analysis. Taken together, our blood cells and hair can give us a safe, reliable reading of our mercury levels.

Faulty metals, faulty behavior. Heavy metals not only damage immunity and physical functioning, but they are also implicated in behavioral and learning disorders. Using hair analysis, researchers found elevated lead and cadmium levels in a group of children with learning disabilities (Pihl and Parkes 1977). Another study found elevations of hair lead and cadmium, as well as calcium and iron, and *low* zinc levels in a group of violent delinquent boys, as compared with the boys' nondelinquent brothers. Hair lead and cadmium were elevated among a group of Maryland schoolchildren who scored low on intelligence tests and school achievement. Of particular interest in this study was that there was a positive correlation between high consumption of refined carbohydrates and high cadmium levels; apparently the consumption of junk food contributed to high cadmium content in the hair (Raloff 1983).

Eating slow-cooked beans and sulfur-bearing foods, such as eggs or garlic, and using supplements provide important protection against heavy metal toxicity. Vitamin C, selenium, zinc, and fiber all help to remove heavy metals from the body (Rosenbaum 1984; Gordon 1983). While dietary acts will remove cadmium, lead, and mercury from the body, only political action will stop the seepage of these toxins at their source.

HIGH FATS MEAN LOW IMMUNITY

For years it has been recognized that high-fat diets are associated with an increased incidence of serious diseases, particularly heart disease, our nation's number one killer. It is now also clear that high dietary fat intake can seriously impair immune functioning.

Cholesterol. Just as it has been difficult to establish the relationship between a high-cholesterol diet and elevated cholesterol levels in the blood, there are also conflicting reports about how dietary cholesterol affects immunity. Laboratory animals who are fed high-cholesterol diets seem to be more susceptible to infection. Macrophages with a high level of cholesterol show a decrease in phagocytic ability. Some studies also suggest that high dietary cholesterol may diminish cell-mediated and humoral immunity. However, most of the studies of the effects of cholesterol on immunity are based on feeding cholesterol to laboratory animals, who do not ordinarily consume it (Rosenbaum 1984).

The situation is clearer concerning the dangers of *oxidized* cholesterol, which has definite immune-suppressing effects. Some cholesterol is normally oxidized in the body, and oxidized cholesterol is also present in fried foods, powdered milk, powdered eggs, and other cholesterol-containing foods that are allowed to stand at room temperature. The oxidized form of cholesterol is a highly reactive *free radical* — a molecular fragment that is capable of damaging the cells, producing genetic damage, and perhaps even causing cancer — and constitutes a threat to your immune functioning. Oxidized cholesterol may also prove to be the real culprit in atherosclerosis and heart disease. These findings should persuade you to avoid fried foods and to store your animal products carefully in sealed, refrigerated containers (Weiner and Goss 1983; Rosenbaum 1984).

Why high-fat diets raise your cancer risk. Strong evidence exists that high-fat diets increase the risk of cancer, particularly of the colon and rectum — the most frequently fatal form of cancer. A high-fat diet leads to elevated levels of *bile acids* in the colon. These break down into deoxycholic and lithocholic acids, which are dangerous carcinogens. Vegetarians have low levels of bile acids in their bowel, and they also have a relatively low rate of colorectal cancer (Vitale 1975). Cancer of the breast, pancreas, gallbladder, ovary, uterus, and prostate, as well as leukemia, are all positively correlated with a diet high in animal protein, fat, and cholesterol (Carroll 1977; Posner, Broitman, and Vitale 1980). High-fat diets and obesity also correlate strongly with the incidence, tumor size, and speed of development of breast cancer (deWaard 1982).

Biological magnification. One of the dangers of a diet high in animal fats is that animal products provide concentrated doses of contaminants, due to a principle known as *biological magnification.* Suppose that a clam absorbs toxic metals from bay mud. Next, a lobster eats a lot of clams and stores an even larger quantity of the toxic chemicals. The lobster then concentrates the toxic chemicals, which would cause the next animal consumer to fall ill from eating too many chemical-containing lobsters. DDT and the immunosuppressive metal mercury are two well-known chemicals that are subject to such biological magnification.

How should this influence your choice of foods? Plants are at the bottom of the food chain. They do not store internally many chemicals that are not necessary for their growth. By washing your vegetables and fruits, you remove a certain amount of unwanted trace chemicals. This is why genuine "organically" grown fruits and vegetables are valued. Being grown without chemical fertilizers or pesticides, this type of produce *is* safer, is definitely "better," and by all means tastes like "real" fruit. Washing simply removes the outer residues of chemicals, leaving potentially harmful chemicals within our average "chemical" crops. Most animals, however, do not wash their food, and hence they consume these chemicals when they eat plants. The farther up the food chain you go, the more likely you are to find unwanted chemicals in organisms; therefore, plant products are generally safer than animal products in terms of their chemical composition.

The dangers of polyunsaturates. There are basically two different kinds of fats, saturated and unsaturated. "Saturated" fats are so called because all of their available carbon bonds are taken up by hydrogen atoms, while "unsaturated" fats have some carbon bonds left free, not attached to hydrogen atoms. Generally the more solid a fat is, the more saturated it is. Animal fats, which are usually solid at room temperature, are generally highly saturated.

Vegetable and fish oils, on the other hand, are generally unsaturated. Because diets high in saturated fats have been implicated as a risk factor in heart disease, there has been a marked increase in the use of unsaturated vegetable oils — such as soy, safflower, sesame, peanut, corn, and sunflower — made from seeds, legumes, and nuts.

Now we must warn that this switch to polyunsaturates can be potentially dangerous. Your diet must contain *some* unsaturated fatty acids for immune protection; deficiency of unsaturated fatty acids inhibits antibody responsiveness (Rosenbaum 1984). However, an *excess* of polyunsaturated fatty acids in the diet of laboratory animals has been shown to produce a profound suppression of immune functioning, manifested in shrinking of the thymus, atrophy of lymphoid tissues, and a depression of cell-mediated immunity and antibody response to antigen challenge. Graft rejection is delayed, and some studies also show a reduction in the ability of certain fighting cells to engulf and destroy bacteria (Rosenbaum 1984).

Polyunsaturated fats undergo a process in the body known as *lipid peroxidation,* a process similar to the development of rancidity in oils. Lipid peroxidation releases dangerous free radicals. Some scientists suspect that the increased use of polyunsaturated fats in our diet is responsible for the high incidence of cancer in Western civilization, since unsaturated fats both suppress immune functioning and perhaps promote the development of tumors (Rosenbaum 1984). In the next chapter, we will describe how antioxidant nutrients can be taken to protect against free radicals.

The more unsaturated a fat is, the more it can harm your immunity. Most vegetable oils are about 80 percent unsaturated. We recommend peanut oil and olive oil, which are only about 50 percent unsaturated, for your cooking needs. Used sparingly in stir frying and salad dressings, these oils will supply the small amount of unsaturated oils required for immune functioning (remember that whole grains and other vegetables also supply some unsaturated oils). Used since antiquity, peanut and olive oils exemplify the dietary wisdom often found in "ancient" foods.

Your wisest approach, in general, is to avoid overconsumption of fatty foods in any form. By shifting your diet away from high-FAT

fat animal products and eating more plant products, you will automatically reduce your exposure to contaminants and increase your intake of the protective nutrients that strengthen your immune defenses. Appendix 3 summarizes the effects of different fats on immune functioning. For definitions of unfamiliar terms, see Table 7 in Chapter 6.

High-protein diets can deplete calcium. Although too little protein in the diet can produce serious immune deficiencies, it is also possible to get too much of a good thing. Americans eat approximately twice the amount of protein required by healthy people. This excessive intake of protein, largely in the form of animal products, can actually be harmful. Animal protein is usually accompanied by a high proportion of saturated fat. Moreover, according to the principle of biological magnification, meat, milk, dairy products, poultry, and fish can all yield concentrated doses of hormones and antibiotics with which the animals have been treated. These substances can seriously disrupt your immune functioning. In addition, meat is rich in phosphorus, and eating too much meat can throw off the calcium-phosphorus balance (which should be 1:1), contributing to calcium loss from the bones and bone weakening. Excess protein may also cause a deficiency of vitamin B_6 — a critical nutrient for immunity and a protective factor against heart disease (Martin and Tenenbaum 1980).

DRUGS

Heavy, habitual use of any drug would logically suppress immune function. Alcohol, caffeine, and tobacco used excessively are potentially harmful drugs, particularly when we are ill or exposed to an infectious agent.

Alcohol. While moderate alcohol consumption (one or two glasses of wine a day) has been shown to be protective against coronary heart disease (Weiner and Goss 1983), excessive alcohol intake leads to blood abnormalities, degeneration of the heart muscle, peripheral neuropathy, muscle disorders, degeneration of the central nervous system (especially the cerebellum and the cerebral cortex), chronic lung disease, malignancies of the head and neck, intestinal malabsorption, low blood sugar levels, liver disease, and increased susceptibility to infection (McLaren 1982).

The intestinal malabsorption caused by alcohol abuse may lead to deficiencies in vitamins B_1, B_2, B_6, B_{12}, folic acid, niacin, vitamin C, magnesium, zinc, and protein (Roe 1976). All of these nutrients but niacin have been shown to play a role in immune functioning.

Alcohol has been known for some sixty years to be associated with an increased risk of cancer, especially of the upper respiratory and gastrointestinal tracts. Why alcohol promotes cancer is not entirely clear. Alcohol per se does not produce cancer in laboratory animals, but other substances in alcoholic beverages may be responsible. More than fifteen hundred different substances are known to occur in wine; and nitrosamines and fusel oil, both known carcinogens, are found in some alcoholic beverages. The nutritional deficiency that often accompanies alcoholism may also play a role in promoting cancer. Alcohol may act as an immunosuppressant (Sandler 1983) and may stimulate free radical production (Crary, Smyrna, and McCarty 1984).

This is not to give you the impression that alcoholic drinks are all bad. In fact in moderation, wine, beer, and the occasional cocktail serve as the front line of stress management for too many healthy people to be rejected altogether. But how do we define "moderation"? The answer is surely cultural and individual. Nevertheless, we are fortunate that the British Medical Establishment has considered this problem and offered their suggestions. One liter of wine, two pints of beer, or seven ounces of alcohol in any twenty-four-hour period is their view of moderation! This may be too high for you — but be relieved to know that in alcohol consumption, as in most things, there are no absolutes.

Coffee and caffeine. It has been much more difficult to assess the adverse effects of coffee and other caffeine-containing beverages than it has been to do so for alcohol. It is known that fibrocystic breast disease is associated with the consumption of foodstuffs containing *methylxanthines* — caffeine, theophylline, and theobromine. These substances are found in coffee, black tea, cola drinks, and chocolate. Susceptible women who eliminate these items from their diet generally feel a rapid improvement in their fibrocystic disease. The methylxanthines act on hormones that cause the fibrocystic nodules to be deposited in the breast.

Coffee is also suspected to play a role in cancer incidence, but this has been difficult to document. Some studies have shown a positive correlation between coffee consumption and cancer of the pancreas, the fourth most common cause of cancer death (Anonymous 1982a). Other studies have implicated coffee as a risk factor in esophageal, kidney, and prostate cancer, although the findings are inconsistent. Caffeine itself is not necessarily the suspected culprit in cancer risk, since decaffeinated coffee drinkers show the same patterns of cancer incidence. Rather, some other constituent(s) in the coffee must be responsible (Sandler 1983).

Since the Western world seems to run on this drug (coffee), relying on its effects for the stimulation needed to keep awake in an increasingly mechanized existence, it may be worthwhile to take a closer look at this reported association between pancreatic cancer and coffee consumption.

Pancreatic cancer has been increasingly appearing over the past few decades, and there is a positive epidemiological association between coffee consumption and the disease in twenty countries. In none of the studies, though, have I seen an evaluation of the effects of what people put in their coffee, the kinds of vessels they drink it from, or the temperature at which it is sipped. Each of these other factors is important and may explain why the evidence is never very strong for pancreatic cancer and the consumption of coffee. It might very well be that those who use cyclamates, or saccharin, to sweeten their coffee are at increased risk, or that the Styrofoam cups so often used in takeout drinks break down into carcinogens in the coffee, or that those who drink their coffee when it is very hot are at some increased risk. Until these cofactors are evaluated, those of us who *must* have our coffee should minimize our risk by following some common sense rules.

First, reduce your coffee drinking to a maximum of three cups a day (the risk goes up above this point). Next, do not use artificial sweeteners. The safety factor of all of these compounds is highly questionable. If you must sweeten, use a natural product such as honey. Next, wait until it has lost its boiling temperature. And last, avoid all plastic containers for hot beverages; there have been some researchers who suspect a chemical reaction with harmful compounds released into the drink.

FOODS THAT CAUSE CANCER

It has been estimated that 35 percent of all cancer deaths are attributable to dietary factors.* (Other cancer death factors are: tobacco, 30 percent; infection, 10 percent; reproductive and sexual behavior, 7 percent; occupation, 4 percent; alcohol, 3 percent; geophysical factors, 3 percent; pollution, 2 percent; medicines and medical procedures, 1 percent; food additives, less than 1 percent; industrial products, less than 1 percent; and unknown factors, 3–4 percent — Doll and Peto 1981.)

Table 4 lists foods that you should *avoid* to minimize your risk of diet-induced cancer. Although it is specifically addressed to cancer prevention, this table serves as a good summary of the general principles of nutritional immunosuppression that we have discussed throughout this chapter. Since cancer is a disease of immune failure, foods that encourage the development of cancer also diminish your immunity on an incremental basis. The more you eat, the more you are "diminished" immunologically.

FOOD ALLERGIES

The foods that depress immunity that we have discussed so far, do so for everyone. For some people, additional allergies to specific foods can be equally disturbing to immune functioning, while other people can eat the same foods with no problems.

If your immune system is constantly being exposed to food allergens and is constantly reacting to them, it is preoccupied with protecting against these invaders. Your immune defenses are thus distracted from their other important functions. In addition, allergic reactions to foods can interfere with digestion and absorption of nutrients, so that even the foods to which you are not allergic are not properly utilized by your body. The results are a reduced nutritional status and a deterioration of immune functioning.

---

*Certainly, *environmental* causes such as air and water pollutants are of great importance in the etiology of cancer. However, by eating nutrient-rich *protective* foods and taking supplements of these nutrients, the environmental forces are somewhat ameliorated.

Obviously, having food allergies is not compatible with maximum immunity. The first step toward eliminating food allergies is to learn to recognize the many symptoms that they can produce. One experienced clinician lists some of the symptoms that cause him to suspect food allergies in his patients:

> Food allergy is suspected when the patient complains of persistent fatigue, puffiness of the face, hands, abdomen or ankles, palpitations (particularly after food), excessive sweating unrelated to exercise, over or underweight and a fluctuation of these and other bizarre symptoms, including emotional and behavioral dysfunction. Digestive disturbances and headache are very common. Often the patient speaks of an intolerance or "opposite reaction" to various medications.
>
> The patient with food allergy may well exhibit the telltale signs of allergy: dark circles under the eyes, stuffy nose causing nasal speech and mouth breathing, watery eyes and a white coated tongue. (Ulett 1980)

If you are troubled with symptoms such as these, you may want to ask your allergist to order an eight-day rotation diet; or you may want to try eliminating a suspect food from your diet for a couple of weeks, and then reintroduce it and see what happens. If you experience the symptoms that you have been suspecting are an allergic reaction, then you may be allergic to that food. Of course you may be allergic to a number of foods, and then you will probably need expert help to analyze the situation.

All foods are not for all people. One man's meat may truly be another man's poison. For those of you worried about yeast infections (candidiasis), the list of foods that contain yeast in Appendix 4 will be helpful. Other commonly allergenic foods are milk, corn, soy, wheat, cottonseed, and egg. (See Table 5.)

Cytotoxic testing for food allergies. You have probably been hearing about the new "cytotoxic tests" for food allergies, and you may be wondering what these tests are and whether they are reliable.

In essence, the method of cytotoxic testing is based on provoking an immune response in your white cells. A blood sample is collected after fasting and prepared for testing. Then small amounts are mixed with samples of food allergens. If your immune system is hypersensitive to a specific allergen, the white cells

TABLE 4
Anti-Immunity Foods

The foods in this table should be *avoided* to minimize your risk of diet-induced cancer and to promote maximum immune readiness.

Food Category	Foods to Avoid
Beverages	Alcohol; cocoa; coffee; flavored and colored beverages; canned and pasteurized juices; artificial fruit drinks; all artificially sweetened drinks; non-dairy creamers.
Dairy products	All processed and imitation butter, ice cream, and toppings; all orange and pasteurized cheeses.
Eggs	Fried.
Fish	Deep-fried.
Fruit	Canned, sweetened.
Grains	White flour products; hull-less grains and seeds (e.g., pasta, crackers, snack foods, white rice, prepared or cold cereals, cooked seeds).
Meats	All red meat products should be reduced and eventually eliminated.
Nuts	Roasted and/or salted, especially peanuts.
Oils	Shortening; refined fats and oils (unsaturated as well as saturated); hydrogenated margarine.
Seasonings	Pepper; excessive use of hot spices.
Soups	Canned and creamed (thickened); commercial bouillon; fat stock.
Sweets	Refined sugars (white, brown, turbinado); chocolate; candy; syrups; all artificial sweets.
Vegetables	Canned; deep-fried potatoes in any form; corn chips.

Additional recommendations: avoid foods that have been sprayed with insecticides, food additives (especially monosodium glutamate [MSG] and others ending in "-ate"), and foods with artificial colors, flavors, and preservatives.

Source: Manner Metabolic Physicians, 1981

in the blood sample will (theoretically) undergo certain changes. Foods that have been identified as allergenic by cytotoxic testing are then eliminated from the diet. The remarkable improvements in symptoms that often result are the most convincing evidence of the accuracy of the cytotoxic tests.

After following a diet that eliminates allergenic foods for some time (perhaps three months), these foods are gradually reintroduced, one by one, into the diet, and tolerance levels established. By avoiding too-frequent exposure to allergenic foods through a careful rotation diet, most people are able to eat these foods without experiencing symptoms.

MALNUTRITION IS THE PROFOUNDEST IMMUNOSUPPRESSANT

To put our concern with disease in perspective, we should understand that the most common cause of immune deficiency among

TABLE 5

Common Foods That Produce Allergy

Food Group	Method of Exposure
Cereals	
Wheat	Inhalation, contact, ingestion
Corn	Ingestion
Rice	Ingestion
Barley	Ingestion
Buckwheat	Contact, ingestion
Vegetables	
Legumes	Ingestion
Soybeans	Ingestion, contact
Fruits	
Banana	Ingestion
Mango	Ingestion
Pineapple	Ingestion
Nuts	
Coconut	Ingestion
Cashews, etc.	Ingestion
Seeds (most highly allergenic food group)	
Cottonseed	Ingestion
Castor bean	Ingestion, inhalation
Mustard seed	Ingestion
Sesame, poppy, caraway, and anise seeds	Ingestion
Beverages	
Chocolate	Ingestion, contact
Coffee (green)	Ingestion, inhalation
Carbonated soft drinks	Ingestion of flavoring and coloring additives
Beer	Ingestion, contact
Yeast and molds	Inhalation
Milk and other dairy products	Ingestion
Meat, fish, and poultry	Ingestion

humans is protein-energy malnutrition. One hundred million children suffer from malnutrition worldwide (particularly in Third World countries), and malnutrition accounts for half the deaths of children before the age of five. The subsistence diets that result in malnutrition usually consist mainly of carbohydrate foods, which may fill the stomach but still do not supply adequate calories (energy). Such diets are also lacking in essential amino acids and other nutrients required to build protein in the body, especially zinc, pyridoxine (vitamin B_6), and folic acid.

Even in our well-fed society, marginal to moderate protein-energy malnutrition is common in innercity ghettos. It also affects more than 15 percent of patients in acute care *hospitals* in this country, owing to a combination of poor diet because of sickness (and poorly designed hospital diets!) and the breakdown of body proteins as a result of the stress of surgery and infection (Rosenbaum 1984). Other people susceptible to malnutrition are cancer patients, the elderly, and infants with low birth weight (Chandra 1981).

Protein-energy malnutrition has characteristic effects on the immune system. Cell-mediated immunity is particularly compromised. The thymus and other lymphoid tissues are more sensitive to nutritional deficits than most other organs and so begin to atrophy at early stages of protein-energy malnutrition. This results in decreased T cell numbers and production (Chandra 1981). Many indicators of humoral immunity may remain unchanged or be increased, but this does not mean that humoral immunity is not also compromised. There are normal numbers of B cells, but there may be increased production of antibody. Serum antibody levels usually associated with allergic responses are much higher than normal.

Secretory IgA (a type of antibody) is often markedly reduced on mucosal surfaces, creating a gap in the first line of immune defense against pathogens; while phagocytes usually show a marked reduction in their ability to destroy bacteria and fungi. The *lysozyme* (a natural bactericide) in tears and saliva is also decreased (Chandra 1981).

With such breaches in their immune defenses, people suffering from protein-energy malnutrition are much more susceptible to bacterial, fungal, and viral infections. They have more frequent episodes of infectious disease, the disease is more severe, and their recovery is much more prolonged (Barrett 1980).

As devastating an immunosuppressant as malnutrition may be, most nutritionally induced illnesses are reversible through supplementation of the deficient nutrients. (In the case of very young children who do not receive adequate nourishment during the critical period of growth, the resultant damage may *not* be reversible.)

Obesity reduces immunity. In the "rich" nations, it is obesity, not undernutrition, that is the most common nutritional disorder. Obese people tend to have more infectious diseases than people of normal weight, and their mortality rate from infection is higher (Rosenbaum 1984). Animal studies have suggested that obesity may be related to autoimmune diseases. Obesity also greatly increases the risk of heart disease and diabetes.

In a study of obese children and adults, about one-third of the subjects showed impairments of cell-mediated immunity and a reduced ability of white cells to kill bacteria. T cell numbers and antibodies remained normal (Chandra 1980a).

It seems that obesity is accompanied by its own peculiar form of malnutrition. For reasons that remain unknown, obese people are consistently found to have deficiencies of zinc and iron, which are responsible, respectively, for T-cell-mediated immunity and phagocytic activity of white cells (Rosenbaum 1984).

It is obvious that the most dangerous food "additive" of all is the excess food that is not necessary for normal functioning. The health problems associated with overeating are far more common than those caused by actual food additives (Sandler 1983).

Now that you know the pitfalls to be avoided in planning your daily diet, let's move on to review the very convincing evidence that specific foods and nutrients can be adjusted and balanced in a total program to enhance your immunity. (To quickly summarize this chapter, review the Avoiding Unhealthy Food Component of the Im.Q. test, reproduced on the next page.)

Avoiding Unhealthy Food Component

Severely restrict fats and meats in diet.	Avoid smoked foods (containing nitrates, nitrites, and erythorbates).	Avoid food chemicals and additives (e.g., colorings and flavorings).
10 pts.	*9 pts.*	*8 pts.*
Avoid white and brown sugar.	Avoid refined white flour baked products.	Avoid deep-fried foods.
7 pts.	*6 pts.*	*5 pts.*
Avoid barbecued foods.	Avoid overeating.	Avoid or limit caffeine to 50 mg per day.
4 pts.	*3 pts.*	*2 pts.*

Your score _____

Maximum score this block _____ 54 _____

∘ 6 ∘
Nutrition for Immunity

PROTECTIVE AND DEFICIT FOODS

As a "food first" nutritionist, I firmly recommend *dietary* sources of nutrients as the primary source. Vitamin/mineral tablets are also recommended but as a secondary source of immune-enhancing nutrients. Assuming we follow the dietary recommendations made in this and other chapters and eat the protective foods, while avoiding as much as possible the deficit foods, how do we know if we are absorbing all of the "good" constituents from our foods and supplements? What if we are utilizing certain nutrients at higher than usual levels? What if we are excreting vitamins at higher than normal rates? In short, how do these very individual parameters of our nutritional needs get quantified?

Fortunately, precise vitamin assays are now possible. Using a new technique (*protozoal assay*), one scientist has made obtaining such analyses a straightforward task for your physician. By drawing a sample of your blood, a distinct vitamin profile can be drawn of your biochemical needs (Baker 1983). Utilizing this technique as well as a hair analysis (which is accurate for toxic metals, questionable for other minerals) and a diet survey of foods eaten, you should be able to see how much of each protective nutrient you are getting down at the cellular level. Then you can adjust your intake of foods and supplements accordingly.

WHAT ABOUT ETHNIC DIFFERENCES?

In an earlier book, *The Way of the Skeptical Nutritionist,* I presented the case for diets based on our ethnic background. My argument was based on a study of the medical-anthropological literature and my travels over a fifteen-year period when I observed, first-hand, the tremendous diversity of human eating habits and diets. It was and is my belief that man has evolved to specific ecological niches primarily by learning to eat foods from those niches that would enable him to survive. Through long periods of time in these specialized food "bowls," each ethnic group has adapted to its own supply and, through a feedback mechanism, *been adapted* to these foods. Perhaps on subtle enzymatic levels, one group is able to eat fava beans, for example, while another group of people develops hemolytic anemia from the same vegetable.

Simply put, not everybody can assimilate the same foods in the same way. Obviously a descendant of an Alaskan Eskimo is different from a Bantu descendant or a Yemenite, even if they all live in New York City and dress similarly, work at similar jobs, drive similar cars, and so on. In our mechanistic age, doctors — even some very excellent "alternative" healers — tend to treat all people as though they were identical. It would be advisable to investigate the ethnic factor in any individualized diet program and compute this element into the final recommendations. While this key element cannot be overlooked, it also can only be approximated at this time and depends to a great extent on the individual's knowledge of his own ethnic and cultural history.

Having outlined several key elements of any nutritional program, we can now look at the relationships between nutrition and immunity.

STIMULATING NATURAL IMMUNITY

You do not need to resort to high technology to stimulate your natural immunity. While genetic engineering laboratories churn out costly interferons to repair the ravaged defenses of the sick, you can *prevent* many immune problems by making wise use of the nutrients we will discuss in this chapter. Here we present the proof, based on extensive research with animals and humans, that familiar nutrients have specific effects on your immune functioning.

Some of these nutrients must be consumed in relatively large quantities of a gram or more a day (such as vitamin C), while others are needed in only trace amounts, expressed as millionths of a gram. But, regardless of the absolute quantity required, your health can be seriously impaired if these substances are not present in the proper amounts and proportions to each other.

You will learn that you may sometimes need to reduce your dosage of some supplements under certain conditions. Even some of the most critical nutrients can sometimes suppress your immune functioning (iron, for example) in the presence of infection.

In this chapter, we will concentrate on the vitamins and minerals with demonstrated specific effects on immune functioning. Research on the immune effects of single nutrients is a very new field. For some nutrients, most of the evidence so far is based only on limited animal studies. The findings are summarized for your reference in Table 6. When the implications for human immunity are clear, we so indicate in our discussion of the individual nutrients.

Research on the immune effects of nutrients is generally reported in technical language. For definitions of unfamiliar terms, refer to Table 7.

Please bear in mind that the supplement ranges mentioned in our discussion of each nutrient are not prescriptions; rather they reflect the dosage range in which the nutrients are commonly taken as supplements.* Supplement requirements vary greatly from one person to the next, reflecting our unique biochemical make-ups. Just because a friend is taking a certain dosage of some nutrient, that does not mean the same dosage is right for you. In setting up a supplementation program, you should consult with a nutritionally oriented practitioner to assess your specific needs and determine what part of those needs will be supplied by your food, and what part by supplemental vitamins and minerals.

---

*Dosage ranges in this book exceed the RDAs. This is consistent with maximizing immune function and is clearly discussed in our earlier books and in the next section.

TABLE 6

Immune Effects of Single Nutrients

	Lymphocytes					Immunoglobulins					Other Immune Functions								
	Lymphoid Anatomy	Total Lymphs in Blood	T and B Cell Differential	Proliferative Response	Splenic PFC Response	Serum Ig Values	Primary Response	Secondary Response	Secretory IgA	Blocking Ig	Delayed Skin Sensitivity	Graft Rejection	PMN Phagocytosis	PMN Bactericidal	Monocyte Function	RES Function	Complement	Inflammatory Response	Host Resistance
Vitamins																			
A Excess	⇑				⇑		N N	⇑			N ⇓	⇑				⇑ N	⇓	⇓	⇑
A Deficit	⇓	N ⇓	⇓↓⇓ N	⇓	⇓			⇑	⇓↓		↓			⇓		⇑		⇓	↓⇓
Thiamin Deficit	⇓	⇓			⇓		⇓					⇓							↓
Riboflavin Deficit	⇓	⇓			⇓		⇓												
Pantothenic Acid Deficit	⇓	N	⇓		⇓↓	↓⇓	⇓												
Pyridoxine Deficit	↓⇓	↓⇓	⇓	⇓	⇓	⇓↓	↓⇓	⇓			↓⇓	⇓				N		⇓	
B$_{12}$ Deficit			↓				N		↑		↓↓	↑							
Folic Acid Deficit	⇓	↓↓⇓ ⇓	⇓			⇓	⇓			⇓⇓	N ⇓ N						⇓	↓⇓
C Excess			⇑	N ⇓	↑		⇑					↑ ⇓					↑	↑ ⇑
C Deficit			⇓ N	⇓		N	N ⇓			⇓	⇓	⇓	N	⇓			↓⇓	
E Excess	⇓		↓⇓	⇑	⇑	⇑	⇑				⇑		⇑ ↓		⇑			⇑
E Deficit	⇓ N			⇓	⇓		⇓								⇓			⇓
Minerals																			
Iron Excess											⇓							↓⇓ ⇓
Iron Deficit	↓⇓ ↓⇓	↓⇓	↓⇓	↓⇓		N	N ⇓		↓		↓	N⇓ ⇓↓	↓	⇓		↑	↓⇓	↓⇓ ↓⇓
Zinc Excess											↓⇓	⇓	⇓	⇓				
Zinc Deficit	↓⇓	⇓	⇓	↓⇓	⇓	⇑	⇑	⇓		↓⇓	⇓↓⇓	⇓ ↓			↓	⇓	↓ ⇓
Magnesium Deficit	⇑			⇓	⇑	⇓	⇑	⇓			⇓ ↑		⇓					⇑
Selenium Excess				⇑		⇑												
Lipids																			
Cholesterol Excess			⇑		↓⇓						⇓			⇓	⇑ ⇓	⇓		⇓
Fatty Acids Excess		⇓	⇓		⇓	⇓					↓ ↓			⇑				⇑
Fatty Acids Deficit		⇓			⇓ ⇓													
Polyunsaturated Fatty Acids Excess	⇑	↑⇓ ↓⇓	⇓		⇓	⇓					↓⇓↓	↓		↓⇑	↓	⇓

Any reported change in immune function (top) associated with nutritional variable (left) indicated by direction and length of arrows. Solid arrows indicate human studies; open arrows, animal findings; N, normal findings; PMN, polymorphonuclear leukocyte; PFC, plaque-forming colonies; RES, reticuloendothelial system.

Source: Beisel et al. 1981

TABLE 7

Indicators of Immune Function

(A Glossary of Technical Terms Used in Reporting Test Results)

Term	Explanation
White cells	
Total T and B cells	Includes both T and B cells
T to B cell ratio	Normally B cells constitute approximately 25% of circulating T and B cells
Splenic PFC response	Response of plaque-forming cells in the spleen which produce antibody
Proliferative response	Ability of T and B cells to respond to stimulation by antigens or mitogens by multiplying
Helper to suppressor ratio	Ratio of T helper to T suppressor cells; normally H:S is approximately 1.8 : 1
Null cells	Immature, as yet undifferentiated, T cells
Natural killer cells	T-cell derived white cells that kill foreign cells directly, by producing cytotoxin (cell poison)
White cell cytotoxicity	Ability of sensitized white cells to attach to and kill target cells
Immunoglobulins	
Antibody titer	Proportion of antibody to antigen
Primary antibody response	Production of antibodies in response to first exposure of the host to a given antigen
Secondary antibody response	Production of antibodies in response to exposure to an antigen with which the host has had prior contact; normally much faster than primary antibody response
Blocking Ig	Antibody that blocks the ability of T and B cells to kill tumor cells
Secretory IgA	Present in saliva and mucosal fluids; first line of defense against invading pathogens and food allergens
IgE	Causes common allergic reactions; also acts against parasites
Phagocytes:	
Chemotaxis (migration)	Ability to be attracted to target area
Motility	Speed with which phagocytes move toward target area; a component of chemotaxis
Opsonization (attachment)	Ability to adhere to a target
Engulfment	Ability to ingest target
Cidal capacity (killing, bactericidal capacity)	Ability to destroy target

Term	Explanation
Other:	
Delayed skin (dermal) sensitivity	Inflammatory response after injection of pathogen or pathogen product
Graft rejection	Ability to reject foreign tissue; while often undesirable in clinical practice, this is a positive indicator of immune functioning
RES function	Immune responsiveness of the reticuloendothelial system — a phagocytic system located in reticular connective tissue of the spleen, liver, and lymphoid tissue
Complement	Series of enzymatic proteins that trigger each other to amplify many immune functions

A NOTE ABOUT DOSAGES, OR WHY THE RDAS DON'T COUNT

The Recommended Dietary Allowances, or RDAs, were established in 1941 in response to the threat of war. They were determined in an effort to define nutrient needs for mass-feeding programs, in which whole populations might need to be supplied with *minimal* diets. These recommendations are now being applied for purposes for which they were *never intended*. They continue to be used as the official guidelines for practically all nutritional enterprises in this country. They are used as the acceptable measure for feeding the armed forces and, of course, are repeatedly quoted by conventional medical "officials" to argue against an increase in vitamin/mineral intake among the general population.

How were these nutrient requirements established? First, the *mean quantity* of a given nutrient that a population requires was determined according to the standard that half the people eating less than this quantity might show *no* signs of deficiency, and that half of those with an intake *exceeding* this quantity may show signs of deficiency. Next, because the mean is an estimate, to allow for variability among individuals the actual RDA is set at two standard deviations above this quantity. This adjustment is supposed to assure that 98 percent of all healthy persons in the American population will have their needs for a particular nutrient satisfied by the amount specified. This amount obviously exceeds by a large margin the *minimal* nutrient requirement for most people in the population. On the other hand, even by the standards used to determine the RDAs, a full 2 percent of the population, or more than four million people, will suffer from a deficiency of some nutrients if they follow the RDAs.

Now, going beyond the question of these figures for our minimal nutrient requirements, we might want to know how much of each nutrient we need for *maximum* nutrition. Based on clinical, epidemiological, and firsthand evidence, the scientists and physicians who are members of several innovative organizations (the Orthomolecular Medical Society, the American Academy of Medical Preventics, the Society for Clinical Ecology, the National Health Federation, to name a few) have noted in their clinical experience that much higher amounts of specific nutrients may be needed to bring some of us to a state of exceptional health. These ranges are those I make throughout this book.

Are these dosages of vitamins and minerals safe? That is the kind of question most often asked whenever the subject is raised at lectures offered to the general public, not yet convinced of the efficacy or safety of large doses of nutrients.

The answer is simple, the reasoning long. In essence, owing to individual differences regarding need, food processing, which destroys many critical nutrients, and newer knowledge, very large dosages of certain nutrients may be beneficial for some people. I have discussed the reasons in a previous book (Weiner 1981) and refer those interested in the details to that and other books such as *Mega-Nutrition,* by Richard Kunin, McGraw-Hill, 1980.

VITAMINS

VITAMIN A

Vitamin A, or retinol, has long been known to promote *nonspecific* resistance to a wide variety of pathogens. This is partly due to its involvement in the production of mucopolysaccharide, a component of the *mucous membranes.* An early sign of vitamin A deficiency is damage to the linings of the respiratory, digestive, and urogenital tracts (Neumann 1977). By helping to preserve the integrity of skin and mucous membranes, vitamin A helps to maintain the protective barriers against infectious organisms entering the body. Vitamin A is also needed for the production of bacteria-fighting lysozymes in tears, saliva, and sweat (Rosenbaum 1984).

Recent research has shown that vitamin A also has a powerful effect on *specific* immune system functions, stimulating both cell-mediated and humoral immunity. Studies of animals with vitamin A deficiency have shown atrophy of thymus and lymphoid tissue, decrease in total number of T and B cells, and depression of T cell response to mitogens and antibody response to infectious agents, including bacteria, viruses, and fungi (Rosenbaum 1984). Vitamin A deficiency increases susceptibility to viral, bacterial, and protozoal infections and makes these problems worse and more often fatal. Other immune system changes associated with vitamin A deficiency include decreased T to B cell ratio, T and B cell proliferative response, spleen cell response, delayed skin sensitivity, monocyte (a kind of white cell) function, and inflammatory response (Beisel et al. 1981; Chandra 1980b; Nauss 1982).

Most studies of the immunological effects of vitamin A have employed laboratory animals with a deficiency of the vitamin. In contrast, a study by Cohen et al. (1979) describes the use of megadoses of vitamin A in humans who had had major surgery (Rosenbaum 1984). As a result of surgery, people often experience a suppression of immune function for weeks, with a decrease in cell-mediated immunity and in macrophage and neutrophil function. This immunosuppression may be a result of the stress related to surgery and/or an effect of anesthesia.

In the Cohen study, patients scheduled for extensive surgery were divided into two groups; one was given large daily doses of vitamin A, and the other served as a control. Blood samples were collected one day before surgery, one day after surgery, and seven days after surgery. The vitamin A treated group showed increased T cell activity seven days after surgery, while the control group showed the usual immunosuppression. Thus vitamin A was shown to be capable of blocking the suppression of immune function that is often associated with surgery.

The patients in this study received very large doses, 300,000 to 450,000 IU, of vitamin A daily for one week after surgery. It is noteworthy that there were no signs of toxicity from these megadoses. When taken in excessive amounts, vitamin A produces a characteristic toxicity pattern of headache, vomiting, vertigo, blurred vision, liver damage, and sometimes yellowing of the skin. In fact, vitamin A toxicity is the most common form of any vitamin toxicity, largely because vitamin A is oil soluble. Whereas water-soluble vitamins are constantly being flushed out of the system, vitamin A can accumulate in the body's fat cells, building up to a level where symptoms appear. Because of the possibility of overdose, many people have shied away from vitamin A, even though the toxicity is easily corrected by reducing the vitamin's intake (McLaren 1982). The absence of toxic symptoms in the above study should help to reassure you of the safety of this important protective vitamin.

Vitamin A appears to be one of the most important protective nutrients against cancer. In studies using animals or human blood samples, various forms of vitamin A seemed to reduce the conversion of altered cells into cancerous cells (Weiner and Goss 1983) and to protect against tumors induced by chemical carcinogens (Chandra 1980b). More recently a study in the Philippines found that high weekly doses of vitamin A and vitamin A precursor helped to protect chewers of betel nut and tobacco leaf from chromosome breaks and oral cancer. Users of these substances have a high rate of oral cancer (Rosenbaum 1984). Vitamin A also appears to be generally protective against the immune-suppressing effects of stress (Rosenbaum 1984).

Green and yellow fruits and vegetables are an important source of vitamin A (in decreasing order, beginning with those highest in vitamin A content: carrots, sweet potatoes, spinach, cantaloupe, apricots, broccoli, peaches, cherries, tomatoes, and asparagus). Milk and milk products, beef liver, and fish liver oil are other sources of this important protective vitamin.

The supplement range is from 20,000 to 100,000 International Units (IU) per day. As a reference point, one medium-size raw carrot contains about 10,000 IU of vitamin A, and one-quarter pound of beef liver contains about 50,000 IU.

VITAMIN B$_1$ (THIAMIN)

This mildly immunity-enhancing B vitamin is involved in appetite regulation, carbohydrate metabolism, blood building, production of hydrochloric acid for digestion, energy, growth, learning capacity, and maintaining the tone of the heart and smooth muscles (Weiner 1981).

Vitamin B$_1$ has less pronounced effects on the immune system than some of the other B vitamins. With thiamin deficiency, there are minor decreases in lymphatic organ size, total number of T and B cells in the blood, spleen cell response, primary immunoglobulin response, delayed skin sensitivity, and host resistance to infection (Beisel et al. 1981).

Foods containing thiamin include peas, lima beans, asparagus, corn, cauliflower, potatoes, watermelon, sweet potatoes, spinach, broccoli, Brussels sprouts, blackstrap molasses, brewer's yeast, brown rice, fish, meat, nuts, organ meats, poultry, and wheat germ.

The supplement range is from 50 milligrams to several grams. Two tablespoons of brewer's yeast contain about 3 milligrams of thiamin, while one cup of sunflower seeds contains about 2 milligrams of this B vitamin.

VITAMIN B$_2$ (RIBOFLAVIN)

Along with other B complex vitamins, riboflavin is involved in maintaining the mucosal barriers that help to defend your body against infection.

Riboflavin is an immunity promoter and is involved in the production of antibodies. Deficiencies are linked to decreases in antibody response, lymphatic organ size, total number of T and B cells in the blood, spleen cell response (Beisel et al. 1981), and inhibition of tumor growth (Posner, Broitman, and Vitale 1980). It is not known whether riboflavin deficiency diminishes cell-mediated immunity.

Other important functions of riboflavin include formation of red blood cells, cell respiration, and metabolism of carbohydrates, fats, and proteins (Weiner 1981).

Foods containing riboflavin include broccoli, spinach, asparagus, Brussels sprouts, peas, corn, lima beans, snap peas, cauliflower, green peppers, blackstrap molasses, brewer's yeast, nuts, organ meats, and whole grains.

The supplement range for riboflavin is 50 milligrams to several grams. One cup of Brussels sprouts contains about 2 milligrams of riboflavin.

VITAMIN B$_6$ (PYRIDOXINE)

Of all the B vitamins, pyridoxine seems to be the most important for proper immune functioning, with deficiencies causing more serious immune problems than with the other B vitamins.

Like some of the other B vitamins, the immunity-enhancing work of pyridoxine begins with the body's external defenses against pathogen invasion, since proper pyridoxine intake is necessary to the health of the mucous membranes.

Pyridoxine is involved in antibody formation, and its deficiencies are associated with diminished antibody responsiveness to antigen challenge (Rosenbaum 1984). With pyridoxine deficiency, there is impairment of T-cell-mediated immunity (Rosenbaum 1984), as well as decreases in thymus size and weight, total number of T and B cells in the blood, T to B cell ratio, white cell proliferative response, spleen cell response, serum IgA values, delayed skin sensitivity, graft rejection, inflammatory response (Beisel et al. 1981), phagocyte chemotaxis (Rosenbaum 1984), and inhibition of tumor growth (Posner, Broitman, and Vitale 1980). Unfortunately, there are no reported studies of the effects of megadoses of this important vitamin.

Besides its role in supporting immune function, B_6 appears to be a key factor in protecting against atherosclerosis and heart disease. When there is a deficiency of pyridoxine, the amino acid methionine is converted in the body to the very toxic chemical homocysteine. Pyridoxine helps to convert this homocysteine to the harmless substance cystathionine; but if there is not enough pyridoxine present, homocysteine accumulates in the blood and causes atherosclerotic deposits to form in the blood vessels. Foods high in B_6 and low in methionine are thus protective against atherosclerosis. These include bananas, avocados, lettuce, carrots, tomatoes, onions, kale, spinach, apples, sweet potatoes, and asparagus, in descending order. Foods high in animal fat and protein are generally the reverse — high in methionine and low in B_6. This may well be the reason why high-fat diets — which are lacking in protective B_6 — are associated with a high incidence of heart disease (Weiner and Goss 1983).

Vitamin B_6, in one of its forms, may also help to prevent clumping of the clot-promoting platelet cells within the blood vessels. Such clumping causes dangerous clots to form, blocking the vessels and leading to heart attack (Weiner and Goss 1983).

Pyridoxine is also involved in hydrochloric acid production for digestion, weight control (through proper utilization of fat and protein), and the ion balance of the nervous system (Weiner

1981). With zinc and folic acid, it is essential for nucleic acid and protein synthesis. Pyridoxine and zinc enhance each other's effects and have similar influences on immune functioning (Rosenbaum 1984).

In addition to the low-methionine fruits and vegetables mentioned above, other sources of pyridoxine include: blackstrap molasses, brewer's yeast, green leafy vegetables, meat, organ meats, wheat germ, whole grains, dried liver, prunes, and peas.

The supplement range is from 50 to 200 milligrams. One cup of peas contains about 2 milligrams of pyridoxine. Vitamin B_2 may be necessary to help produce the form of B_6 that restores immune functioning after a deficiency state (Rosenbaum 1984).

VITAMIN B_{12} (CYANOCOBALAMIN)

Because it is not possible to induce vitamin B_{12} deficiency in laboratory animals, and humans with a deficiency of this vitamin *alone* (untreated primary pernicious anemia) are very rare, most of the information about its effect on immune functioning comes from observations outside the body (in vitro). According to a Japanese study (Sakane et al. 1982), B_{12} may exert a regulatory influence on T helper and suppressor cells.

Other studies suggest that cobalamin stimulates immune functioning, with a deficiency leading to decreased T and B cell proliferative response, white blood cell phagocytosis and ability to kill bacteria, and an increase in blocking immunoglobulins (Beisel et al. 1981).

Along with folic acid, vitamin B_{12} is involved in the synthesis of the hemoglobin in red blood cells. It also contributes to appetite, cell longevity, health of the nervous system, and metabolism of carbohydrates, fats, and proteins (Weiner 1981).

Cobalamin is found in cheese, fish, milk and milk products, organ meats, cottage cheese, and eggs.

The supplement range is from 50 to 100 micrograms. One-quarter pound of beef liver contains about 90 micrograms of cobalamin.

FOLIC ACID

Folic acid is an immunity-enhancing member of the vitamin B complex, with deficiencies leading to suppression of both cellular and humoral immunity — as observed in laboratory animals and in humans suffering from a form of anemia due to folic acid deficiency.

Specific immune functions depressed by folic acid deficiency include: lymphatic organ size, T to B cell ratio, T and B cell proliferative response, spleen cell response, primary and secondary immunoglobulin responses, delayed skin sensitivity, white blood cell phagocytosis, inflammatory response, number of T cells in lymphatic organs, host resistance to infection (Chandra 1980b; Beisel et al. 1981), and inhibition of tumor growth (Posner, Broitman, and Vitale 1980).

Along with vitamin B_6 and zinc, folic acid stimulates nucleic acid and protein synthesis. It affects appetite, body growth, reproduction, hydrochloric acid production, and red blood cell formation (Weiner 1981).

Foods containing folic acid include green leafy vegetables, milk and other dairy products, organ meats, oysters, salmon, brewer's yeast, dates, tuna, and whole grains.

The supplement range is from 400 micrograms to a few milligrams. One cup of steamed spinach contains 448 micrograms.

PANTOTHENIC ACID

This B vitamin is found in so many foods that dietary deficiencies are rare. Pantothenic acid is an immunity enhancer, promoting antibody formation. Animals with an artificially induced pantothenic acid deficiency showed decreased production of antibodies in response to antigen challenge by bacteria or viruses. The vitamin appears to promote antibody release from plasma cells (Rosenbaum 1984).

Pantothenic acid deficiency is also associated with decreases in lymphatic organ size, T to B cell ratio, spleen cell response, serum immunoglobulin levels, primary and secondary immunoglobulin responses (Beisel et al. 1981), and inhibition of tumor growth (Posner, Broitman, and Vitale 1980). A deficiency of pantothenic acid has no known adverse effect on cell-mediated immunity (Beisel 1982).

Besides its role in immune functioning, pantothenic acid is involved in metabolism of carbohydrates, fats, and proteins; growth stimulation; and the utilization of other vitamins (Weiner 1981).

Brewer's yeast, legumes, organ meats, salmon, wheat germ, whole grains, mushrooms, and elderberries all contain pantothenic acid.

The supplement range is from 50 milligrams to several grams. One cup of cooked mushrooms contains 82 milligrams of pantothenic acid.

VITAMIN C (ASCORBIC ACID)

When Nobel laureate Linus Pauling first announced that high doses of vitamin C helped to prevent or lessen the severity of viral diseases such as the common cold and influenza, the public rushed to stock up on this nutrient. Researchers, seeking to verify or disprove Pauling's claims, generally did not use the high doses recommended by Pauling; but even at dosages of less than one gram a day, most workers found that vitamin C reduced the severity of viral upper respiratory illnesses. Orthomolecular practitioners, using doses of at least 10 grams of vitamin C a day, report even greater benefits in reducing the symptoms of bacterial and viral diseases. Nor is it just minor illnesses such as the common cold and flu that are influenced by vitamin C. According to case studies by Dr. Robert Cathcart and Dr. Russ Jaffe, this vitamin, when taken in a balanced nutritional program, also speeds recovery from mononucleosis, viral pneumonia, and even some cases of AIDS!

Surprisingly, vitamin C deficiency has no apparent effect on most parts of the immune system, including the thymus and other lymphoid tissues, the T and B cells, and the antibodies. The beneficial immunological effects of vitamin C seem to be due to its enhancement of phagocytic functions — specifically, its stimulation of the motility of macrophages and neutrophils. This very specific effect of vitamin C has been confirmed by a study involving subjects with Chédiak-Higashi syndrome, a condition in which the neutrophils have low motility. Vitamin C was able to stimulate neutrophil motility in these people at the relatively low dose of 200 milligrams a day. To a much more limited extent, vitamin C may also have an influence on the ability of phagocytes to kill bacteria and fungi (Rosenbaum 1984).

It remains a mystery how vitamin C improves our immunity against viruses. The vitamin appears to have no direct antiviral effect when examined outside the body. Recent studies suggest that vitamin C may stimulate T and B cell transformation, which means the vitamin does have an effect on cell-mediated immunity and may help explain its antiviral properties. If vitamin C enhances T cell function, it may also promote the release of interferons, which attack viruses (Rosenbaum 1984).

One of the most exciting areas of vitamin C research is its therapeutic use in treating cancer. Drs. Linus Pauling and Ewan Cameron, a Scottish cancer surgeon, have reported that a dose of 10 grams a day is beneficial in some cancer cases, while Robert F. Cathcart III, M.D., uses much higher doses. According to Dr. Cathcart, the more serious the illness, the more vitamin C we need. Proper dose is determined by giving increasing amounts of ascorbic acid up to the point where diarrhea occurs, and then reducing the dosage by 10 percent. The dosage at which the bowel symptoms are produced is known as the *bowel tolerance level* (Cathcart 1981). In the case of cancer, proper dosage can be as high as 100 grams a day (Cathcart 1984).

How does vitamin C fight cancer? Since macrophages are believed to play a critical role in fighting tumors, the macrophage-stimulating properties of vitamin C would help to explain its beneficial effects. Moreover, the vitamin's stimulation of T cell transformation would help increase the antibody response to the tumor and stimulate the production of T killer cells, which destroy cancer cells (Rosenbaum 1984).

Aspirin has an anti-vitamin C effect, promoting the loss of vitamin C through the urine and also decreasing uptake of the vitamin by white blood cells. Taking aspirin also seems to increase the danger of a spreading viral infection, as has been observed in Reye's syndrome in children (Rosenbaum 1984). For these reasons, you may want to think twice before taking aspirin along with vitamin C for your cold or flu.

In its role as an antioxidant and free radical scavenger, vitamin C further helps to fight cancer by preventing the formation of carcinogens in the body. For example, ascorbic acid inhibits the formation of nitrosamines by reacting with nitrite before the nitrite can combine with amines in the diet to form the highly carcinogenic nitrosamines (Newberne and Suphakarn 1983). As an antioxidant, vitamin C protects against lipid peroxidation, preventing the formation of dangerous free radicals (Germann 1977). It has a synergistic effect when taken with other antioxidants: the more vitamin C you take, the less vitamin E you need. '

In helping to combat the adverse effects of stress, vitamin C helps to counteract the immunosuppressive effects of corticosteroids, yet at the same time assists in the anti-inflammatory function of the steroids (McCarty 1982).

Besides its specific effects on immune functioning, ascorbic acid is also critical to bone and tooth formation, collagen production, and other forms of tissue integrity. Thus this vitamin is essential in maintaining your body's external defenses against infection (Neumann 1977).

Dietary sources of vitamin C, beginning with those highest in vitamin C concentration, are: green peppers, broccoli, Brussels sprouts, cauliflower, strawberries, spinach, oranges, cabbage, grapefruit, cantaloupe, and papaya. Because your body may require much higher amounts of vitamin C than can be obtained from food alone, Dr. Pauling and many other proponents of this amazing vitamin advocate daily consumption of a vitamin C supplement as a protective measure.

The supplement range is from 1 to 4 grams, on up to bowel tolerance when ill. CAUTION: Do *not* self-prescribe this vitamin as a *substitute* for professional treatment in the case of serious illness. Consult your health professional for diagnosis and advice about vitamin therapy as well as other treatment.

VITAMIN D

Vitamin D is the only vitamin that we are able to manufacture ourselves. This internal synthesis requires sunlight, and not everyone is exposed to enough sunlight throughout the year to maintain adequate levels of calciferol in the body from this source alone. For this reason, many people take vitamin D supplements.

Because vitamin D is fat soluble, it is stored in the body's fat cells. The vitamin is added to animal feed, and so we consume it in our meat. It is also added to enriched milk products and flour (Gordon 1983).

Although vitamin D is an essential nutrient, it is possible that too much vitamin D might actually suppress immune functioning.

Although vitamin D deficiency has been found to decrease phagocytic ability (Chandra 1980b), according to another study, the vitamin may also have an immunosuppressive effect that helps to regulate immune processes. In a study at the Scripps Clinic, in La Jolla, California, vitamin D was shown to suppress the production of *interleukin-2* by human white cells. Interleukin-2 stimulates the formation of T helper and suppressor cells and antibodies, and so by reducing interleukin-2 production, vitamin D functions as an immunosuppressant. It may be that vitamin D works to prevent excessive white cell proliferation. Malignant B and T cells, as well as activated T cells, have been observed to contain receptors for this vitamin.

This study suggests that *for people who already have suppressed immune systems, it would be unwise to take vitamin D supplements* (Rosenbaum 1984).

It is not surprising that vitamin D has immunosuppressive effects, since it has the structure of a steroid hormone. Other steroid hormones, such as corticosteroids and progesterone, are also immunosuppressive.

But, vitamin D has many essential functions in the body and must not be completely eliminated. It plays a key role in forming bone through its regulation of calcium and phosphorus metabolism; it helps to regulate heart action, maintain the nervous system, and promote normal blood clotting, muscular contractions, and skin respiration (Weiner 1981). Vitamin D along with calcium may also help to prevent the bone degenerating effects of corticosteroids (McCarty 1982). However, *excess* vitamin D may also promote the creation of harmful calcium deposits in the blood vessels.

Natural sources of vitamin D, besides sunlight, include egg yolk, organ meats, bone meal, and fish.

The supplement range is from 50 to 500 IU. One cup of milk contains 100 IU of calciferol. CAUTION: Vitamin D supplementation is *not* recommended for people with reduced immune functioning.

VITAMIN E

Hailed in recent years as a "miracle vitamin," vitamin E is best known for its antioxidant properties. It is much less recognized for its ability to stimulate the immune system and to protect against infection.

Adding extra vitamin E to the diet of animals has been shown to significantly enhance their ability to produce antibodies in response to pathogen exposure. Giving vitamin E in conjunction with selenium enhances the immune-boosting effects even further (Rosenbaum 1984).

Most research on nutrients investigates the effects of deficiencies. Vitamin E deficiency has been shown to result in decreased lymphatic organ size, T and B cell proliferation, white blood cell function, inflammatory response, and host resistance to infection (Beisel et al. 1981). In the case of vitamin E, much more work has been done on the effects of larger than normal doses, rather than on artificially created deficiencies. Elevated levels of vitamin E, in addition to producing enhanced antibody response, have been observed to improve white cell bactericidal activity, phagocytosis, and host resistance (Beisel et al. 1981). Dietary supplements of vitamin E enhanced T helper cell activity in mice (Tanaka, Fujiwara, and Torisu 1979), and vitamin E supplements may also help to reduce the immunosuppressive effects of corticosteroids (McCarty 1982).

Vitamin E is a powerful antioxidant that prevents the formation of free radicals and protects cell membranes against lipid peroxidation. These antioxidant and free radical scavenging properties help to protect against cancer in a variety of ways. For example, vitamin E helps to block the formation of carcinogenic nitrosamines out of nitrites in foods. In animal studies, vitamin E, added to food or applied to the skin, decreased the severity and number of tumors produced by carcinogenic substances (Newberne and Suphakarn 1983).

In the process of killing bacteria, *macrophages produce free radicals.* High doses of vitamin E, as well as the antioxidant mineral selenium, help to protect macrophages from damage by these bactericidal free radicals (Crary, Smyrna, and McCarty 1984).

The antioxidant properties of vitamin E also protect the lungs from air pollution damage (Chandra 1980b).

Among its other important properties, vitamin E protects against dangerous blood clots and affects blood cholesterol levels, blood flow to the heart, strength of capillary walls, and muscle and nerve maintenance (Weiner 1981). It protects against stress in general, and some forms of vitamin E seem to increase fertility in laboratory animals.

Vitamin E is found in dark green vegetables, eggs, liver and other organ meats, wheat germ, vegetable oils, oatmeal, peanuts, and tomatoes.

The supplement range is from 100 to 1200 IU. One tablespoon of wheat germ oil (a very rich source) contains 40 IU of vitamin E.

MINERALS

COPPER

Copper deficiency has been linked to lowered resistance to infective challenge (Beach, Gershwin, and Hurley 1982) and shortened survival time and greatly increased mortality following infection (Chandra 1980b). Copper deficiency in conjunction with protein deficiency has been shown to decrease the resistance of rats to salmonella bacterial infection and may do the same in humans. Copper may also protect against cancer. In studies with animals, copper supplementation has been shown to result in fewer liver tumors (Beach, Gershwin, and Hurley 1982). Copper deficiency reduces the activity of the form of *superoxide dismutase* (SOD) — an important antioxidant — that is dependent on copper and zinc (Crary, Smyrna, and McCarty 1984). But an excess of copper has been shown to impair host resistance and antibody response (Beisel 1982).

Copper is involved in body healing processes, bone formation, hair and skin color, and red blood cell and hemoglobin formation.

It is found in oysters, legumes, nuts, lecithin, organ meats, seafood, raisins, molasses, and bone meal.

The supplement range is from 2 to 5 milligrams. One cup of soybeans contains 2 milligrams of copper.

IRON

Of all the minerals and vitamins, iron is one of the most likely single nutrients to be deficient in the absence of any other form of malnutrition (Beisel 1982). Iron deficiency is common among premenopausal women worldwide, as well as among malnourished children.

Because iron is required to produce the hemoglobin that carries oxygen to all the body's cells, as well as to promote resistance to stress and disease, people worry that they may be iron deficient and often take this mineral as a supplement. As we will explain, *too much iron sometimes may be just as dangerous as too little.*

The body has several mechanisms for maintaining iron levels within the appropriate range. Both deficiency and excess of iron can cause immune problems, and both increase the danger of infection (Rosenbaum 1984).

Iron deficiency, because it decreases the availability of oxygen to the body's cells, can have an adverse effect on the cells of the immune system, since their oxygen requirements are relatively high. Depending on the severity of the iron deficiency, there may be atrophy of lymphoid tissues and a decrease in the total number of T and B cells in the blood. Other immunosuppressive effects may include decreased responsiveness to antigen challenge, reduced inflammatory response, and reduction of delayed skin hypersensitivity reaction (Beisel et al. 1981; Rosenbaum 1984). Iron deficiency impairs the ability of phagocytes to kill bacteria, thus impairing resistance to infection.

Excessive levels of iron in the body are also immunosuppressive, resulting in reductions in macrophage phagocytosis and increased susceptibility to many kinds of infections (Beisel et al. 1981). Most microbes require iron in order to reproduce, and so it is critical to prevent pathogens from obtaining iron. When an infection is present, a number of defense mechanisms are set in motion to make iron *unavailable* to the micro-organism. For example, the white blood cells secrete a chemical that lowers blood iron and also causes a fever. Elevated body temperature makes it more difficult for bacteria to absorb iron (Rosenbaum 1984). This is why it is important *not* to take that multivitamin mineral pill when you are ill. You do not need that added iron.

It is also important to remember that *iron supplementation can increase the dangers of infection,* especially among people suffering from malnutrition. Before such individuals can benefit from iron supplementation, their nutritional status, and especially their protein levels, must be raised so that they can use iron properly rather than leaving it available to any micro-organism that happens to invade their bodies.

Cancer cells, too, need iron, and the body has several ways of withholding iron from cancer cells. People and animals with excessive iron levels tend to have an increased risk for developing cancer, and the tumors are often associated with the site where the iron is deposited in the body! Besides nourishing cancer cells, excess iron may also suppress the cancer-killing function of the macrophages and interfere with T and B cell activity (Weinberg 1983).

A brilliant epidemiologist looked at two hundred years of cancer case histories in which "hopeless" cancers were cured when severe bacterial infections developed. The study hypothesizes that the cancers may have been cured partly because the bacteria depleted the body's iron supply, producing a reactivation of the immune system and killing the tumor cells (Martin 1984).

Excess iron is also suspected to be involved in the pain, swelling, and joint destruction of rheumatoid arthritis. Iron-deficient populations in Third World countries are rarely affected by rheumatoid arthritis (Martin 1984).

Because of the dangers associated with iron excess, it is a good idea to get your iron from foods. Spinach, lima beans, peas, Brussels sprouts, artichokes, broccoli, cauliflower, strawberries, asparagus, snap beans, blackstrap molasses, eggs, fish, organ meats, poultry, wheat germ, desiccated liver, and shredded wheat all contain iron (Weiner 1981; Germann 1977).

The usual supplement range is from 15 to 50 milligrams. One large shredded wheat biscuit supplies 30 milligrams of iron. CAUTION: For people with infections or malnutrition, iron supplementation may not be advisable.

MAGNESIUM

Although magnesium is known to be critical in regulating many vital body functions, a deficiency of this mineral has not been shown to produce any major impairment of immune functioning in humans.* In animals severe and prolonged magnesium deficiency causes the immune system to overreact, with overproduction of certain white cells and excess release by the mast cells

---

*However, it has recently been determined that deaths from toxic shock syndrome occurred due to *magnesium loss* brought about by tampons, which absorbed this vital mineral!

of chemical mediators, which cause a rise in serum histamine (Rosenbaum 1984).

A survey of the literature reports equivocal findings concerning the immune effects of magnesium deficiency, including increased lymphatic organ size but decreased spleen cell response, serum immunoglobulin levels, primary and secondary immunoglobulin responses, graft rejection, and host resistance to infection (Beisel et al. 1981).

Magnesium deficiency has been found to be associated with increased cancer risk in both humans and laboratory animals. Magnesium-deficient diets are related worldwide with an increased risk of esophageal cancer, and magnesium deficiency seems to promote various forms of cancer in rats. It may be that magnesium deficiency is not the *cause* of cancer, but rather part of a larger pattern of mineral imbalance.

Magnesium is unquestionably a critical nutrient for other purposes. It is involved in the body's acid/alkaline balance and in the metabolism of blood sugar to produce energy. It also regulates the metabolism of calcium and vitamin C (Weiner 1981).

Because our eating patterns have changed so radically within the last half century, most people who consume the typical Western diet are at risk for a borderline magnesium deficiency. This is partly due to a sharp increase in dietary phosphorus from meats, preserved foods, soft drinks, and other sources. Excess phosphorus can bind other important minerals, such as magnesium, zinc, and copper, and make them unavailable for digestion. Thus high phosphorus intake increases the need for magnesium (Gordon 1983).

Excess phosphorus intake also necessitates the use of balancing calcium supplements; but excess calcium can contribute to calcification of the arteries and heart problems. To avoid these problems, magnesium supplements should be taken along with calcium, preferably in a ratio of 1 to 1. Unfortunately, many calcium/magnesium supplements on the market are in the ratio of 2 parts of calcium to 1 of magnesium, and hence may aggravate the problems of excess calcium (Gordon 1983).

Magnesium-rich foods include honey, bran, green vegetables, nuts, seafood, spinach, bone meal, and kelp.

The supplement range is from 300 to 500 milligrams. Remember that if you are taking a calcium supplement, ideally you should use an equal dosage of magnesium. One cup of roasted peanuts (with skins) contains 420 milligrams of magnesium.

MANGANESE

Little is known about the effects of manganese on the immune system. Manganese deficiency has been found to lead to decreased antibody synthesis and/or secretion, and supplemental manganese in animals' diets has led to improved antibody production. However, substantial excess manganese levels *inhibit* antibody formation, T and B cell stimulation, and chemotaxis of T and B cells. Manganese is known to induce mutation in cells and is a proven carcinogen in mammals (Beach, Gershwin, and Hurley 1982).

Like vitamins C and E, manganese functions as an antioxidant and may help to counteract the immunosuppressive effects of corticosteroids (McCarty 1982). It is a component of one form of the antioxidant superoxide dismutase (Crary, Smyrna, and McCarty 1984).

Manganese is involved in enzyme activation, reproduction and growth, hormone production, tissue respiration, vitamin B_1 metabolism, and the utilization of vitamin E (Weiner 1981).

Bananas, bran, celery, cereals, egg yolks, green leafy vegetables, legumes, liver, nuts, pineapples, and whole grains are all sources of manganese.

The supplement range is from 5 to 50 milligrams (Weiner 1981).

SELENIUM

Research on the immunological effects of selenium began only recently in Western countries; much of the earlier work was done in the Soviet Union and Eastern Europe. Soviet researchers report that selenium promotes humoral immunity in a manner similar to vitamin E, and that the two in combination work synergistically. A sodium salt of selenium given to laboratory animals increased their antibody response to a variety of antigens. Selenium also potentiates the ability of phagocytes to kill bacteria and increases the capacity of macrophages and related cells to kill tumors (Rosenbaum 1984).

Selenium also fights cancer by protecting against carcinogens. In fact it is the most potent known broad-spectrum anticarcinogenic agent (Crary, Smyrna, and McCarty 1984). In animals exposed to various carcinogens, tumor incidence has been shown to be greatly reduced when the animals are given supplementary selenium (Newberne and Suphakarn 1983).

A powerful antioxidant, selenium protects cell membranes from lipid peroxidation and prevents the release of free radicals. Like vitamin E, it protects macrophages from destruction when they release free radicals to kill bacteria (Crary, Smyrna, and McCarty 1984). It may also help to counteract the immunosuppressive effects of corticosteroids, while at the same time aiding their anti-inflammatory effects (McCarty 1982).

Selenium is extremely valuable for treating poisoning with heavy metals such as mercury and cadmium, since it facilitates their excretion from the body. Of course these toxic metals have immunosuppressive effects in their own right.

While selenium deficiency can have adverse effects on the immune response and other bodily functions, too much selenium can also be dangerous. Selenium is highly toxic in excess dosage, producing symptoms such as loss of hair and nails, dizziness, fatigue, and dermatitis. However, some recent reports indicate that high-dose supplementary selenium was tolerated over long periods without toxicity. Organic selenium, in the form of *high-selenium yeast,* is less toxic than sodium selenite, and the organic form may generally be safer to use at high doses (Crary, Smyrna, and McCarty 1984). Nevertheless, until we know more about dosage, we recommend that you exercise great caution in using selenium supplements. If you think you are not obtaining sufficient selenium from your diet, a careful supplement regimen can be worked out. Remember that selenium levels in the soil vary greatly, and so the foods raised on these soils will have varying selenium contents.

Foods containing selenium include butter, smelt, wheat germ, apple cider vinegar, garlic, asparagus, and fish. Low-fat foods from the meat group, breads and cereals, and legumes are good sources of this vital mineral. However, because soil levels of this nutrient may vary, eating a broad spectrum of the above foods is advised.

The supplement range is from 10 to 100 micrograms. CAUTION: Selenium is highly toxic in overdose!

ZINC

Zinc is an extremely important immune stimulant specifically promoting T cell immunity. People suffering from severe protein-energy malnutrition usually do not have adequate intake of zinc, and it is mainly because of this zinc deficiency that malnourished people show a severe depression of cell-mediated immunity, leaving them highly susceptible to infection (Rosenbaum 1984).

Zinc deficiency can produce atrophy of the thymus gland and a reduction in the number of mature T cells. As a result, many cell-mediated immune functions are impaired, including delayed skin sensitivity, graft rejection, T and B cell bactericidal activity, and natural killer cell activity (Beach, Gershwin, and Hurley 1982; Rosenbaum 1984). The T helper to suppressor ratio may also be decreased. In addition, zinc deficiency leads to poor healing of burns and other wounds (Chandra 1980b), further opening the way for infection.

Humoral immunity is much less affected by zinc, although it does promote antibody production that is dependent on T helper cells (Rosenbaum 1984).

Besides its role in promoting immunity, zinc is essential for many other bodily functions. It is required for the production of some eighty enzymes in humans, as well as nucleic acid and proteins (Rosenbaum 1984). It is involved in carbohydrate digestion, growth and development of sex and reproductive organs, the sense of taste, and the metabolism of vitamin B_1, phosphorus, and proteins (Weiner 1981).

Knowing how important zinc is, it is a cause for concern that the average American diet may not be supplying adequate amounts of this critical mineral. To make the situation even worse, other factors can deplete zinc levels further, including overconsumption of bran and certain other high-fiber foods, cadmium toxicity from tap water, and alcohol abuse. Zinc deficiency can be especially dangerous for children and pregnant women, who require zinc to promote rapid growth (Rosenbaum 1984).

It is no wonder that many people are taking zinc supplements today. But now we must sound a caution, because there is another side to zinc's influence on immune functioning. While zinc promotes T cell immunity, it significantly decreases phagocytic immunity. Zinc has been shown to depress the function of neutrophils and macrophages, inhibiting their motility, chemotaxis, and bactericidal and phagocytic abilities (Rosenbaum 1984; Beisel et al. 1981).

The practical implication of this fact is that it may be unwise to use zinc supplements when there is a danger of bacterial infection or when infection is already present. Also, although zinc is known to promote wound healing, it may not be a good idea to use zinc after surgery or burns, since it may encourage bacterial infection. Excess zinc may also promote the growth of the yeast candida, since macrophages and neutrophils are essential for fighting candida infections (Rosenbaum 1984).

Thus, while supplemental zinc may be beneficial in treating T cell immune deficiencies, it can be harmful in the case of bacterial infections. The double-edged sword of zinc's immune effects is an excellent example of why you must be very careful about how you use supplemental vitamins and minerals.

Including zinc-rich foods in your diet will provide you with the protective benefits of this important mineral. Brewer's yeast, liver, seafood, soybeans, spinach, sunflower seeds, and mushrooms are all good sources of zinc.

The supplement range is from 15 to 50 milligrams. CAUTION: Do not take extra zinc when you have a bacterial (or candida) infection, unless advised by your physician.

PROTECTIVE FOODS

Taking vitamin and mineral supplements alone is not enough to ensure optimal immune protection. You also need to consume nutritious foods to supply you with the proteins, carbohydrates, and fats your body requires. Besides providing energy, protein, vitamins, and minerals, certain foods contain protective factors that further enhance your immunity and often specifically defend against cancer.

FIBER

Fiber is well established as a major protective factor against cancer of the colon and rectum, coronary heart disease, appendicitis, hemorrhoids, diverticulosis and diverticulitis, and many other diseases. While it does not appear to have a direct stimulating effect on the immune system, fiber speeds the removal of toxic waste materials in the colon by promoting rapid transit of the stool through the bowel. High fiber intake also seems to promote the presence of beneficial, aerobic (oxygen-using) bacteria in the intestine and to suppress anaerobic (non-oxygen-using) bacteria, which are potentially harmful since they have the ability to break down bile acids into carcinogenic substances. In these two ways, fiber contributes to preventing colorectal cancer.

There are several different kinds of fiber, with different protective benefits. Cereal bran and other sources of cellulose seem to have the most significant effect on the size and transit time of stool. The fibers from fruits and vegetables, on the other hand, seem to have a cholesterol-lowering property.

Some foods with very high fiber content are: almonds, apricots, blackberries, bran breakfast cereals, Brazil nuts, chick peas (garbanzos), coconut, dates, filberts (hazelnuts), figs, guava, loganberries, parsnips, peaches, peanuts, peas, pecans, raspberries, soybean flour, walnuts, whole wheat flour, wheat germ, and puffed wheat (Germann 1977).

Many people eat wheat bran on a daily basis to ensure an adequate fiber intake. In this case once again, it is possible to overdo a good thing. Bran contains phosphorus compounds known as *phytates,* which can form complexes with mineral nutrients and prevent their uptake by the digestive system. Among the minerals that complex with phytate are copper, iron, magnesium, manganese, and zinc (Weiner 1981). Thus, too many phytate-rich foods in the diet can lead to deficiencies of these important nutrients, many of which are known to be important to immune functioning. Zinc deficiency, in particular, is associated with depression of T cell immunity. Among malnourished populations that subsist on grain products, phytate levels are often high in the diet, making immune-protective minerals unavailable and producing an even more profound, immunosuppressive deficiency state.

FOODS AGAINST CANCER

No common, edible vegetable or fruit has been implicated in any type of cancer. On the contrary, we know that certain plant foods are definitely protective against cancer, based on animal research and on studies of the diets of cancer patients. The cruciferous vegetables — Brussels sprouts, broccoli, cauliflower, cabbage, and turnips — contain several substances that protect against carcinogens, induce protective enzyme activity, and suppress free radicals. Several researchers have found that a regular diet of cruciferous vegetables reduces the risk of developing cancer and that the more of these vegetables consumed, the lower the cancer incidence (Weiner and Goss 1983). Spinach, celery, lettuce, and dill also have been found to promote anticarcinogen enzyme activity (Germann 1977). Other protective foods include high-fiber fruits and vegetables and those rich in vitamin A, which has antioxidant and anticancer activity, as noted above.

Other foods, including many components of traditional ethnic diets, may have similar anticancer properties, which may help to explain why some populations have lower cancer incidence than others. It has been found that water extracts of six species of edible mushrooms demonstrated antitumor activity in mice (Ikekawa et al. 1969).

Laminaria, a brown seaweed commonly consumed in Japan, seems to act as a breast cancer preventative in Japanese women, perhaps due to its high fiber content (Teas 1983).

Since immune failure is such an integral part of some cancer development, proper nutrition is obviously an important defense against this much feared disease. Immune processes, which are influenced by nutrition, are involved in the elimination of cancerous and precancerous cells (McBean and Speckmann 1982). Moreover, proper dietary management can play a crucial role when cancer actually does develop — a fact that is all too often overlooked in cancer treatment programs. Cancer patients have specific nutritional imbalances that, if corrected, might greatly enhance their chances for recovery or for longer useful lives by restoring proper immune functioning.

Table 8 summarizes the foods you should emphasize in your diet to minimize your risk of diet-induced cancers. Like its com-

TABLE 8

Pro-Immunity Foods

The foods in this table are recommended for promoting optimal immunity and for minimizing your risk of diet-induced cancer.

Food Category	Recommended Foods
Beverages	Herb teas (e.g., Mathake,* chamomile, mint, papaya; no caffeine); fresh fruit and vegetable juices.
Dairy products	Raw milk; yogurt; butter; buttermilk; nonfat cottage cheese; uncolored cheese.
Eggs	Poached or soft boiled.
Fish	Fresh white-fleshed; broiled or baked.
Fruit	All dried (unsulfured), stewed, fresh, and frozen (unsweetened).
Grains	Whole grain cereals, bread, muffins (e.g., rye, oats, wheat, bran, buckwheat, millet); cream of wheat; brown rice; whole seeds (sesame, pumpkin, sunflower, flaxseed).
Meats	Gradually reduce.
Nuts	All fresh, raw, or lightly roasted (unsalted).
Oils	Cold-pressed oils; olive, peanut.
Seasonings	Herbs; garlic; onion; rosemary; parsley; marjoram.
Soups	Any made from scratch (e.g., salt-free vegetable, chicken, barley, millet, brown rice).
Sprouts	Especially wheat, pea, lentil, and mung.
Sweets	Pure, unfiltered honey; unsulfured molasses; pure maple syrup (in limited amounts only).
Vegetables	All raw and not overcooked, fresh or frozen; potatoes, baked or boiled.

*A Fijian herb long utilized to stimulate immune reactivity, only recently introduced to the West.

Source: Adapted from Manner Metabolic Physicians, 1981

panion Table 4 in the previous chapter, it can be interpreted broadly as a map to guide you toward a pro-immunity diet.

WHAT IS THE IMMUNITY VALUE
OF YOUR DIET?

The two Im.Q. blocks reproduced on the next two pages, taken together, integrate the information contained in this chapter. The Healthful Food Component has been designed to meet most ethnic and individual needs. Interestingly, most ethnic diets, no matter the country, rely on a high fiber, low animal fat, fruit, and vegetable structure. Applied broadly, you should be able to eat in restaurants, on airplanes, or of course, at home while meeting the goals set out in these blocks. An immune-enhancing diet, together with a reasonable amount of vitamins and minerals as supplements, is your key means of raising your resistance against disease, providing you also follow the guidelines of the "mind" and "physical exercise" chapters.

Healthful Food Component*

Eat high-fiber diet (e.g., more than 25 g per day).	Eat moderate-fiber diet (15 to 24 g per day).	Eat foods with anti-oxidants (e.g., fruits and vegetables rich in vitamins A, C, E, and selenium).
10 pts.	*9 pts.*	*8 pts.*
Eat seafood 3 times per week.	Eat whole-grain products.	Drink immune-stimulating herbal teas (Pau D'Arco, Mathake†).
7 pts.	*6 pts.*	*5 pts.*
Eat 25% of daily foods in raw state.	Eat chemical-free foods (i.e., organically grown and processed).	Drink 8–16 oz. freshly squeezed juices (varied) daily.
4 pts.	*3 pts.*	*2 pts.*

Your score _____

Maximum score this block _____ 45 _____

* Score only one fiber cube, whichever is higher.
† Both kinds are particularly effective against candida infections.

The Vitamin and Mineral Component

Daily take:
beta-carotene
  (vitamin A) –
  15 mg (equiv.
  to 25,000 IU)
vitamin C – 2 g
vitamin E – 400 IU
selenium
multivitamin/mineral
  supplement.
 	
10 pts.
	Daily take
	  zinc supplement.
	
	9 pts.
		Daily take
		  calcium/magne-
		  sium supplement.
		
		8 pts.

Daily take
  vitamin B complex
  (50–100 mg).
 	
7 pts.
	Daily take
	  lecithin supple-
	  ment.
	
	6 pts.
		Daily take
		  pantothenic acid
		  and niacin supple-
		  ment.
		
		5 pts.

Daily take
  PABA (a subtle
  B vitamin)
  supplement.
 	
4 pts.
	Every other day take
	vitamin C and
	a multivitamin
	(*without* iron).*
	
	3 pts.
		Every third or fourth
		day take vitamin C
		and a multivitamin
		(*without* iron).*
		
		2 pts.

Your score _____

Maximum score this block _____ 49 _____

* Score one of last two cubes *only* when first 10-point maximum cube is unchecked.

· 123 ·

∘ 7 ∘

The Soma of Motion

OR THE LONELINESS OF THIS
LONG-DISTANCE JOGGER

I REMEMBER THE DAY I stopped jogging. For fear of a heart attack, I had taken up cross-country running in the back of the wooded valley where I live. By jumping over streams and panting up grades for about two miles, you come to a remarkable waterfall. It seemed perfect — in the beginning.

But the loneliness of this long-distance runner began to speak in clear terms. An inner "voice" began to demand, "Stop ... I can't take this anymore." Having been schooled in self-denial from the cradle, I of course attempted to override this inner "weakling." But the more *I* persisted, the louder *it* became!

As time progressed, I faced a genuine crisis. I began to believe this inner argument would lead to a nervous collapse and somewhat regretfully ended my deerlike dashing.

It was a time of great stress in my life, and I came to realize (*years* later) that this running, while good for my muscles, was keeping me *away* from people: and it was people I needed more than running alone to regain my psychic equilibrium.

To compensate for not running, I bought a new bicycle and took to riding it vigorously each morning one mile in the *opposite* direction from the valley — *toward town* and my daily dose of mail at the post office. This substituted for the running, and with other relaxation techniques (including lying on a sofa with a novel each day, drinking passionflower herbal tea, and taking megadoses of certain vitamins and minerals), I learned to calm the inner debate that had threatened to drown me in madness!

The point I am trying to make here is that one form of exercise (in this case running) may not suit the nature of all people. And this may be true at different periods in our life. We may love running at one time, but not at another. Adaptation sometimes requires listening to your inner voice(s)! Doing so may be unfamiliar, even terrifying — but it is the only sure way to determine *your individual needs* for exercise.

I will never understand why we swing so wildly: first we are the most sedentary people on earth, only to become the most obsessed with running! Where is the balance, the *harmony*, instilled by a quiet walk or feeding pigeons in a park?

To gain or regain equilibrium through motion, a more balanced approach than is presently being pursued seems to be indicated.

Having said this, let's see how immunity is enhanced through *moderate* but *persistent* physical activity.

THE SOMATOPSYCHIC BENEFITS OF EXERCISE

Earlier, we spoke of psychosomatic influences on immunity — that is, mind over body. Exercise can be shown to exert a "body over mind," or a *somatopsychic,* effect on the mind, which in turn can influence the immune system to function at optimal levels.

The most direct evidence of a relationship between motion and immunity comes from studies with the obese. We know that unhealthy medical conditions occur more frequently among the overweight, conditions such as gallstones, diabetes, heart disease, and infections. Obesity itself may not be directly causal, but a relationship exists. Why? Specific markers of immune function *are* affected by obesity.

For example, a decreased capacity to destroy bacteria by neutrophils accompanies human obesity (Palmblad et al. 1976). This could be due to certain food factors. Obese people who ate a lot of dairy protein were seen to die more frequently from *lymphomas,* or tumors of the lymph tissue (Cunningham 1976 in Ader 1981). A reduction in dairy protein was seen to be associated with decreased numbers of "certain animal tumors, in mortality/morbidity in viral diseases, and in resistance to bacteria" (Good, Fernandez, and Yunis 1976, in Ader 1981).

How fats, another food component, affect immunity is also interesting. Cholesterol and free fatty acids are known to decrease phagocytosis, and raised cholesterol levels in humans weaken the formation of antibodies and also reduce the proliferation of white blood cells (Ader 1981).

Since obese people often have abnormal blood fat profiles, it is reasonable to state that motion, in reducing obesity and normalizing blood lipids, enhances immunity.

These studies with the obese are a step along the path of understanding how motion affects immunity. What you can do to improve your disease profile is our next topic.

One further note about types of physical motion is in order. "Exercise" generally connotes a certain briskness of action as in jogging or tennis. But this is a peculiarly Western notion of what is capable of stimulating our healing powers. By understanding the Eastern view of physical motion and experimenting with some of those forms of "exercise," you may untap a new joy in physicalness, instead of feeling it is something to get over with, as so many wrist-watching joggers seem to feel.

The new "exercises" now being taught are developed out of Eastern models. Aerobic conditioning, flexibility training, isotonic-isometric-isokinetic conditioning, and various dance-based techniques are all novel methods for moving the inner powers of healing.

PREVENTION AND CONTROL OF DISEASE

With heart disease our number one killer today, exercise has gained increased recognition as an important factor in health promotion. Regular exercise clearly has been demonstrated to be an important factor in controlling cardiovascular disease. It strengthens the heart and lungs, improves circulation, reduces blood pressure, increases the blood's ability to dissolve clots, regulates the concentration of fats in the blood, and reduces the demand on the heart muscle at any level of exertion (Pelletier 1979, 1981).

People who exercise regularly have a greatly reduced incidence of heart attack and other cardiovascular disorders. For example, in a study of active and sedentary postal workers in London, it was found that those who delivered mail had a considerably lower incidence of heart attacks than did those with desk jobs. When these workers died, of various causes, autopsies revealed that the sedentary workers had cardiovascular pathology equivalent to mail carriers ten or fifteen years older (Leaf 1973).

Exercise has long been used as a specific therapy for other diseases as well. About 600 B.C., the Indian physician Sushruta used exercise in the management of certain types of diabetes (Thomas 1981). Still part of the recommended treatment program for many diabetics today, exercise is known to reduce blood glucose levels (Laube and Pfeiffer 1977).

People with asthma also benefit from regular exercise, even those who suffer from exercise-induced asthma. For them, swimming may be the most beneficial activity (Thomas 1981).

Regular, vigorous motion also seems to help prevent osteoporosis, or the loss of calcium from the bones that comes with aging, especially among women. Among the various communities in the world where people are reputed to live well past one hundred, strenuous activity is a way of life. Among isolated groups of centenarians in the Caucasus, for example, physical examination revealed healthy bones among the very elderly (Leaf 1973).

Supporting such findings is the experience of our American astronauts, who under conditions of weightlessness and physical inactivity have been found to suffer a calcium loss from their bones (NAS 1972).

PSYCHOLOGICAL BENEFITS

There is a wealth of information on the effects of motion on the mind. As one researcher summed it up: "The body's influence on the mind can be just as important as the mind's influence on the body. Tension is both mental and physical; and relaxation or relief of tension can be brought about by both mental and physical measures" (Rathbone 1976).

In Chapter 4, we saw that chronic, unresolved stress is one of the great enemies of healthy immune functioning. Unrelieved stress produces corticosteroids, which directly suppress the immune response, and leads to a wide variety of stress-related diseases that further compromise immunity.

Anything that can help to alleviate the build-up of chronic, unrelieved stress must be embraced as a life-saving tool. Exercise is clearly such a stress reliever.

The acquisition of athletic skills and development of physical fitness have been shown to reduce anxiety levels. Such stress reduction may stem from many different aspects of athletic activity — improved self-image, physiological changes in the brain, the process of confronting and overcoming a challenge, and participation in a group activity (Thomas 1981). The lesson here is: rather than sit and watch a sporting event on TV, go out and participate in one!

Although exercise is known to lower anxiety temporarily, stress levels have been observed to rise again a few hours after exercise (Bahrke 1981). However, by reducing anxiety on a daily basis, regular exercise may prevent the development of a pattern of chronic stress that can lead to physical and physiological illness (Morgan 1981).

Vigorous exercise is known to increase the levels of *endorphins,* the morphinelike brain hormones that can produce a sense of well-being and are believed to be responsible for the placebo response. Perhaps because it stimulates endorphin production, jogging is being used as an effective therapeutic tool in many cases of anxiety and depression. Some therapists even jog alongside their clients, providing "talk therapy" between breaths!

If you are a regular exerciser, you can confirm for yourself the observations of researchers that exercisers exhibit less anxiety, tension, depression, and fatigue and have more vigor than people who do not exercise (Blumenthal et al. 1982).

The body can have a powerful influence on the mind. When you are sick, you feel mentally dull and sluggish. When you engage in regular, vigorous physical activity, you generally feel alert and positive. Whenever you are feeling tense, or depressed, your best remedy may be to get your body in motion!

THE DANGERS OF OVEREXERCISE

We cannot urge you to engage in regular exercise without recommending intelligent caution at the same time. The experiences of world-class athletes provide an interesting perspective on the dangers of overdoing a good thing.

Why do athletes get sick? Curiously, research has shown that serious athletes are *not* the healthiest people around. In fact, strenuous training may make athletes more susceptible to illness, depleting the body's energy reserves to the point where the immune system suffers. Strenuous exercise reportedly may aid the development of hepatitis, and in extreme cases may even cause death (Jokl 1977). Therefore, athletes may not be good models for an exercise or motion program, because of their willingness to be "used up."

Besides the effects of training itself, international competition brings athletes into physical contact with a wide variety of people and unusual sources of infection. Athletes who travel frequently may experience jet lag, which disrupts their sleep/wake cycle and imposes extra stress. Unfamiliar foods and waters may make them sick. On Olympic teams, gastrointestinal and respiratory infections are the most frequent medical complaints, with skin infections the next most common (Jokl 1977).

Among women athletes, especially those engaged in marathon running and other grueling tests of endurance, low percentages of body fat can cause hormonal imbalances. Many female long-distance runners, with body fat content far below average, have been observed to suffer a cessation of menstruation or profound irregularities in their menstrual cycles. Because the female hormone system is interrelated with the immune system, there may be an accompanying imbalance in immune functions as well.

Heart attacks in runners. While regular exercise is known to promote cardiovascular fitness, remember that each of us is an individual, and we must all know our personal limits. Too many runners have collapsed with heart attacks in long-distance races for us to approach such athleticism without due caution. There has been much speculation among exercise physiologists about why long-distance runners, who are presumably in good physical condition, suffer heart attacks. One theory is that an improper training diet, along with the loss of minerals through sweating, produces an electrolyte imbalance that results in disturbances of the nerve impulses that pace the heartbeat. (Such drinks as Gatorade were developed to replace these electrolytes and vitamin C for those engaged in strenuous athletic activities.)

The death of runner Jim Fixx from a heart attack provides another perspective. Fixx initially took up running to counteract his known heart disease. Unfortunately, he did not change his high-fat diet at the same time. Fixx's death is evidence that exercise *alone* is not sufficient protection against heart attack — especially in an already compromised system. It must be accompanied by a proper diet.

The lesson is clear: *you should not overexercise an underprotected body,* which has not been supplied with the proper nutrients to support physical exertion. Lengthening one or two legs of a tripod will simply tip it over; the same goes for maintaining a *complete* program of exercise, nutrition, and psychological well-being. These three functions support one another, but they must all be pursued consciously — and conscientiously.

CHOOSING MOVEMENT FOR BETTER HEALTH

With the above cautions in mind, we can now provide some general guidelines for exercising or "moving." No single plan will be right for everyone, and we recommend that you experiment with different activities to find out what you enjoy doing the most. Exercise should benefit both the body and the mind, and if you do not *enjoy* what you are doing, you are defeating half the purpose. Remember the loneliness of this long-distance runner!

If you are overweight, out of shape, or physically infirm, or if you are over forty and have not been exercising regularly, do *not* begin an exercise program without some sort of supervision or advice from a qualified person (for example, a doctor or athletics instructor).

To receive maximum benefits from your exercise program, you must do it regularly — preferably at least six days a week. A well-rounded program is not limited to only one kind of exercise, but should include the following three kinds of physical activity.

Aerobic exercise. Engage in regular, *vigorous* exercise (within your own limits) to improve the function of your heart and lungs and increase your endurance. Such exercise might include, for example, running or brisk walking, swimming, aerobics, bicycling, rowing, rope jumping, or trampolining. You should do this vigorous exercise at least three times a week. You don't need to do the same exercise each time; you may enjoy alternating among various aerobic activities.

Strengthening exercise. Building your muscular strength and tone will protect you against injury and help compensate for the disappearance of strenuous exertion from our modern lives. Weight training (either free weights or machines), calisthenics, swimming, aerobics, most sports, and physical labor all help to build muscle strength; a professional trainer can help set up a progressive program suited to your capabilities. Exercises for strength should be done three times a week, with a day's "recovery period" in between to let the muscles rest and consolidate their gains.

Flexibility exercise. Increasing your flexibility makes you feel better both physically and mentally. It promotes circulation, nerve function, and other bodily processes, thereby improving your overall health. Stretching exercises and yoga are good ways of increasing flexibility. We recommend that you do such exercises daily. Remember to stretch gently; forcing your muscles and joints past their limits can result in injury.

Be sure when you exercise, to do gentle stretching or other *warm-up exercises* before engaging in vigorous activity, to increase the blood supply to the muscles and make them more pliable. This simple precaution will help prevent injuries. At the end of exercising, again allow for a few minutes of *cool-down activity*, such as easy walking, to help the circulation return to normal. Without cool-down exercise, you may experience dizziness or nausea after a period of vigorous activity.

Remember that regular exercise is an end in itself, a break from your other daily activities. Don't feel you must be competitive in your exercise, even against yourself. Accept your exercise time as a period of re-creation, in which you recharge your physical and mental batteries.

Moderation is the key. If the activity you choose is too easy, you will not realize any benefit. If it is too strenuous, you may be doing yourself more harm than good. Allow yourself to get pleasure from your exercise; don't use it as a way of punishing yourself for your past sins. Remember, the better you feel about yourself, the better your immune system is likely to function.

IMMUNOLOGICAL ROGUES
ALSO NEED EXERCISE

Mark Twain used to joke that he got his exercise by walking to the funerals of his more athletic friends! Funny, yes, but *not* a prescription for health and longevity. The same is true with Norman Cousins's reported remission from a fatal illness by watching Abbott and Costello comedies on television. People love that anecdote. What they fail to remember is that Mr. Cousins also took massive doses of vitamins, especially vitamin C, along with his prescription for laughter.

The point is that half-truths are useful for avoiding a commitment to immune enhancement that takes some doing. Mark Twain may have walked (not run) to his friends' funerals, but what else did he do to maintain his equilibrium, and therefore his immunity? Certainly his writing was one such "balancing" factor, but there were no doubt other health enhancing factors that have gone unreported. Regarding exercise, as with other elements of maximum immunity, you may hear that a certain long-lived person got there by drinking, eating, and lazing around, and that therefore fate or genetics is more important than anything we can do. Don't believe it! There may be, in fact, a few great indulgers who live on in years; but they are the exception, not the rule. I call these people "immunological rogues," and by my reckoning they all could have lived to the age of Moses (120 years) had they built upon their fine inheritance with the principles of diet, mind, and exercise I have outlined here.

To review *your* activity level in the Im.Q. game plan, the Exercise Component block is reproduced on the next page.

Please note that when we refer to the word "vigorously," we also mean the completeness of the activity. You need not run or train as an athlete might to score a maximum of 10 points on this block.

The Chinese elders who awaken like flowers each dawn with their T'ai Chi movements are never seen to move abruptly or too quickly. Yet they do their version of "exercise" completely. Likewise with a yoga program. Again, abrupt or vigorous motion is alien to this form of physical cultivation.

The key to deciding what a maximal motion plan is may be

contained in the following words, which I noticed in the window of a neighborhood women's fitness club: "Warm up with us . . . tap the natural energy source within."

The key is to light the inner fire on a daily basis and keep it glowing, without burning down the temple.

Exercise Component: Choose One!

Exercise vigorously and completely* 7 times per week. *10 pts.*	Exercise vigorously and completely 6 times per week. *9 pts.*	Exercise vigorously and completely 5 times per week. *8 pts.*
Exercise vigorously and completely 4 times per week. *7 pts.*	Exercise vigorously and completely 3 times per week. *6 pts.*	Exercise vigorously and completely 2 times per week. *5 pts.*
Exercise vigorously and completely once per week. *4 pts.*	Exercise vigorously and completely occasionally. *3 pts.*	Beginning an exercise schedule. *2 pts.*

Your score _____

Maximum score this block _____ 10 _____

* "Completely" stands for the idea of balance in exercise and includes varied activities, stretching, breathing completely as in yoga, strength work as in weightlifting, maintaining aerobic capacity, etc.

PART III

DISEASE AND IMMUNITY

Overview

IMMUNE DISORDERS
THROUGHOUT THE LIFE CYCLE

No matter what your age and physical condition, you have undoubtedly experienced several immune disorders in your lifetime. Diseases of immune failure can be as disastrous as a crippling autoimmune illness or as negligible as the common cold.

Your immune defenses may be breached at any time in the life cycle. In fact, since some immune disorders are genetic in origin, they can begin as early as the moment that the sperm unites with the ovum. In some rare cases, the result can be a devastating immune deficiency disease, in which the infant is born with absolutely no immune protection.

Even a normal infancy presents prodigious challenges to the immune system. Some infants develop allergies to specific foods, including their mother's milk. Many children are susceptible to allergies not only to foods, but also to pollens, molds, and other environmental substances.

In childhood, also, comes the onslaught of *pathogenic diseases* — mumps, measles, chicken pox, and many others. In the past, such infectious diseases proved fatal to many youngsters. Today immunization has eliminated their dangers; however, side effects have reopened thinking regarding the universal administration of such immunizations.

The autoimmune diseases most typically make their appearance in adulthood, during a person's thirties, forties, or fifties. (A suspected autoimmune form of diabetes, insulin dependent diabetes mellitus, generally appears during youth and is one exception to this statement.)

Having survived the threat of these possible forms of immune failure, the mature adult may still fall prey to cancer, second only to heart disease as a cause of death today.

Of course all these categories of immune failure can occur at *any* age; children do develop cancer, and some adults do catch "childhood diseases" such as mumps or German measles.

Chapter 8 will survey some of the ways in which the immune system can malfunction. Following that we will look at some of the specific diseases that can result from such breakdowns. This survey is not meant to be exhaustive, but to discuss *representative examples* of immune disorders. Some will be very familiar to you, while others may strike you as strange and exotic. Where possible, brief capsule highlights of treatment, both conventional and "alternative,"* will be presented.

You will probably be impressed by the tremendous variety among immune disorders and the many different ways in which they express a breakdown of immune functioning. As you begin to understand the ways in which your immune system is vulnerable to attack, you will see how proper stimulation is a critical line of defense. By following the parameters of maximum immunity described throughout this book (particularly Part II), you should be able to reduce your risk of developing many immune disorders.

ARE ALL DISEASES RELATED TO IMMUNITY?

At times in this book, you may come to the conclusion that the authors believe *all* the ills that man is heir to are related to the immune system! For the purposes of this book, only a few categories of diseases that are clearly related to immune failure are discussed. These are certain pathogenic diseases; cancer; AIDS; the autoimmune diseases; some immune deficiency diseases; candidiasis; and the allergies.

It is true that some researchers go much further in their categorization of immune-related diseases and include heart disease, the aging process itself, Alzheimer's disease, and a legion of others. Only time will bring to us the links that make such suppo-

---

*"Alternative" medicine, for the purposes of this book, will be limited to the effects of various nutrients on immune function. Experimentally, nutrient/immune reactions are appearing in the core of medical literature, the journals. This is not yet so for other "alternative" modalities of treatment, such as homeopathy, acupuncture, herbalism, and so on. When these data appear, new books on immunity will follow.

sitions strong enough to categorize these, and perhaps other diseases, as related to immune failure.

Please do not form the impression that we are offering "cures" for the diseases we discuss in Part III. We do feel, based on clinical, epidemiological, and common sense evidence, that the immune system is responsive to stimulation. However, we do not offer any treatment directions, our recommendations being *suggestive only, not prescriptive.*

○ 8 ○

What Makes Immunity Fail?

SO FAR we have been talking about the immune system in an idealized manner, showing how it works to protect against a wide variety of foreign agents. Yet we all know from personal experience and from observing other people — from the minor suffering of a common cold to the mysterious symptomatology of the autoimmune diseases, from a seasonal case of hay fever to life-threatening cancer — that our natural defenses are often breached.

BODILY DEFENSES

Before we concern ourselves with what goes wrong with the immune system, let's take a look at what kinds of physical defense mechanisms we have — those that a pathogen (disease-causing agent) must overcome or elude before it can cause us any problems. There are both "external" and "internal" defense systems.

External defense mechanisms. The first obvious external barrier is the skin. This layer of tissue encasing our bodies is only about one-twentieth of an inch thick, but it is a highly effective barrier to most pathogens. Not only is the skin relatively impenetrable, but the acidic nature of sweat and other sebaceous gland secretions on the body's surface helps to repel bacteria and fungi.

Another external barrier (although it may not seem external) is the mucous membrane that lines the respiratory and digestive

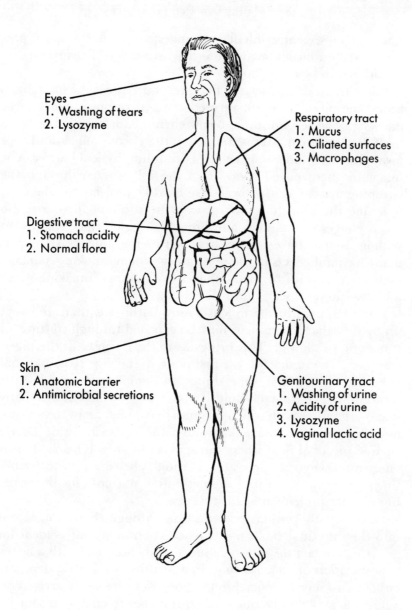

Eyes
1. Washing of tears
2. Lysozyme

Respiratory tract
1. Mucus
2. Ciliated surfaces
3. Macrophages

Digestive tract
1. Stomach acidity
2. Normal flora

Skin
1. Anatomic barrier
2. Antimicrobial secretions

Genitourinary tract
1. Washing of urine
2. Acidity of urine
3. Lysozyme
4. Vaginal lactic acid

Fig. 3. SOME EXTERNAL DEFENSE MECHANISMS

tracts. You see, any inhaled or ingested pathogen must pass through the mucous membrane defenses before it can truly be considered to be *in* the body.

In the respiratory tract, the first line of defense is the small hairs lining the nose; these are very effective at trapping fairly large particles. The second, more comprehensive, defense is the *mucus* itself. Particulate matter is trapped in the viscous mucus and kept away from the underlying cells by this fluid physical barrier. The mucus is then moved away from the cell surface through the sweeping activity of the protective hairlike projections (the *cilia*) that line the bronchial passageways. In addition there are also macrophages in the lungs and bronchial region that swallow up pathogens that have become trapped in the mucus. Among its many harmful effects in the respiratory system, smoking damages both the cilia and the macrophages in the lungs, breaking down the physical defenses against disease.

What happens to the mucus-bound pathogens that are swept up by the cilia? The mucus may be expelled through spitting, or it may be swallowed. This brings us to the defenses in the digestive tract. The stomach is the first place in the digestive tract that is hostile to invaders — the throat and esophagus provide little protection. The stomach fluid is highly acid, which destroys any micro-organisms with which it comes in contact. Some organisms, however, are able to sneak through the stomach inside poorly chewed pieces of food where the acid is not able to reach. This is one reason why complete and thorough chewing (ten to twenty times per small mouthful) is so essential, not only for digestion, but also for protection against disease.

Once a pathogen has passed safely through the stomach and into the intestinal tract, it has reached an area that is ideal for growth — in fact the intestines are already occupied with a heavy concentration of bacteria that, in a healthy digestive system, are either neutral or beneficial to the host. But, the newly arrived organism is at a disadvantage when it comes to competing for resources. Not only is there competition, but some of the resident bacteria also produce antibiotic-like substances as part of their by-products, making the environment even more difficult for newcomers.

The urinary and reproductive tracts also contain external defense mechanisms, including the acidity of their fluids and the presence of lysozyme, an enzyme that is effective against some types of bacteria. Lysozyme is also found in large quantities in tears. Contagious conjunctivitis, or "pink eye," and urinary tract infections seem to be caused by the types of bacteria that are resistant to lysozyme.

The eyes are also protected through their constant washing by tears. The tears are transported through a duct into the back of the throat, where pathogens are subject to the digestive system defense mechanisms.

A pathogen may manage to get past such external defenses any number of ways. It may be carried in, for example, through a puncture wound; that is why puncture wounds are much more dangerous than superficial cuts. It may hitch a ride in uncooked or poorly chewed food, or it may fight its way in with its offensive weapons — which will be described in more detail toward the end of this chapter.

Internal defenses. Once the pathogen is inside, the body has additional defenses waiting. Most of the internal organs are surrounded by a tough membranous *capsule,* which is more resistant to penetration than the organ tissue it protects. Another inherent protective factor are macromolecules (very large, chainlike molecules) in the blood that have antibacterial or antiviral properties. One of these molecules, called glycoproteins, may surround viral organisms and prevent them from reaching a target cell and causing infestation. There are also iron-bearing protein molecules in the blood that compete with bacteria for the iron the bacteria require for growth and reproduction. And of course, we also have our friends the B and T cells roaming the body trying to take care of anything that may have gotten by all these defensive barriers.

Other factors in resistance. Unfortunately, these defense mechanisms do not work equally well in everybody. There are several modifying factors that can influence the efficacy of the body's defenses:

> It is obvious that the external and internal defense forces do not function at the same level of efficiency in all individuals. It is generally recognized that such factors as race, sex, nutritional status, hormonal influences, age, climate, fatigue, and alcoholism markedly influence the level of a person's natural resistance. . . . Blacks

and whites have a different susceptibility to several infectious diseases. For example, blacks are more susceptible to tuberculosis but more resistant to diphtheria and influenza than are whites. (Barrett 1980)

In all the various immune-related disorders, the white blood cells are either absent or insufficient. These protector cells and their functions may be inhibited by a wide range of factors. These include "poor" genes, drugs, radiation, surgery, traumatic injury, malnutrition, stress, and hormonal imbalances.

To see how the immune system is sometimes breached and what kinds of diseases follow, we can look at those organisms that are most familiar to us — the viruses, bacteria, and parasites.

HOW VIRUSES, BACTERIA, AND PARASITES EVADE THE IMMUNE SYSTEM

A pathogen is an organism or a substance that produces disease. The immune disorders we have discussed so far are largely manifestations of something going awry inside the immune system itself. In the case of pathogenic diseases, it is always possible to point to an outside, causative agent — those unseen "bugs" that we were told in childhood swarmed over our unwashed hands. Not all pathogens are invisible, however. Disease-causing organisms range in size from the microscopic virus to very large parasites, and they use a variety of means to by-pass your immune defenses.

Even though pathogenic diseases are associated with specific organisms or their toxic products, the presence of the organism alone is never enough to produce the disease. There must be a breach in your immune defenses in order for the pathogen to take hold and make you ill. This is why, in the middle of an epidemic, some people become sick and others stay healthy. It is not merely a matter of whether you are exposed to the pathogenic organism, but also how well you are able to resist it. Fortunately, we are learning more and more about what we can do to raise our resistance to pathogenic organisms by improving immune functioning.

Disease-causing organisms range in size from the virus, which is so small that a powerful electron microscope is needed to see it, to the tapeworm, which reaches several feet in length at maturity. How does this variety of life forms evade our external and internal defenses? Beginning with the smallest pathogens and working up to the largest, we find a diverse array of mechanisms for eluding the immune system. In the survey of pathogenic diseases that follows, we will first discuss the ways that the immune system defends against each type of pathogen and how that pathogen gets past these immune defenses. Then we will describe some representative illnesses caused by these classes of disease-producing organisms.

VIRUSES

Existing at the very borderline of life, viruses cannot reproduce on their own, but rather must use the reproductive capacities of other organisms. When you have a viral infestation, the viruses actually take over the cells of your body to serve their own reproductive purposes. The immune system has a variety of tactics for controlling a virus, some of which are directed against the body's infested cells. As we know, the T cells can secrete cytotoxins, which kill the infected cells. If a cell is killed before the virus has completed its reproduction, the virus in the cell is also eliminated. Another weapon to keep the virus from reproducing is antibody from B cells, which prevents the virus from attaching itself parasitically to the body's cells. In addition, the antibodies IgM and IgG may themselves serve as killers of virus-infested cells.

T cells participate in the control of viruses in another way also, by secreting lymphokines. One well-known class of lymphokines is interferon, which is being investigated as a weapon against viruses and even cancer. Lymphokines are substances that call macrophages into the fray; the macrophages then phagocytize the viruses directly. Antibodies from B cells also help to promote phagocytosis.

Viruses have an unpredictable way of slipping through our defenses that is known as *antigenic drift*. This means that the organism undergoes random mutations over time that result in its losing antigens that were previously characteristic and acquiring new ones in their place. This makes it very difficult for the immune system to recognize the invader as the same organism that attacked before. It is because of antigenic drift that our immune systems never seem to be prepared for influenza pandemics that come through our area.

To by-pass the body's immune defenses, the influenza virus is able to parasitize the mucous membranes in the outer part of the respiratory system, keeping the virus outside the major stronghold of the immune system. Other viruses, such as herpes, become established in a host cell and then spread to new cells derived from the infested cell, without ever leaving the protective environment of the host cell. Thus the virus is able to reproduce and proliferate safely within host tissue until it is ready to attack.

VIRAL DISEASES

A tremendous variety of diseases are caused by viruses, and many different viruses may all produce similar symptoms. We will now review some representative viral illnesses.

The common cold. The common cold is anything but common. More than one hundred different strains of viruses are able to produce the symptoms that we recognize as a cold — sore throat, sneezing, runny nose, cough, and general malaise. Even if your system has encountered, and is prepared to repel, fifty different types of cold virus, you are still susceptible to at least another fifty variations on the theme. Although a cold can make you feel miserable for a few days, this type of viral infection is obviously extremely mild compared to the severity of some of the other viral diseases.

Influenza. Several types of viruses also cause influenza. The viruses involved have a tendency to mutate into different forms, which the immune system recognizes as entirely different organisms. If the immune system has not been exposed to the precise antigenic configuration of a mutated virus, even if it was easily able to recognize the earlier form, it must manufacture new antibodies to counter the attack.

For most people, influenza is a decidedly unpleasant experience, with runny nose, cough, sore throat, headache, and muscle and joint aches, but it is one from which they recover without problems. However, influenza *can* lead to viral pneumonia and other complications that might prove fatal, especially among people who are already debilitated.

Measles. This extremely contagious viral disease used to be part of the growing-up experience of practically every child. Now that measles vaccine is widely available, there has been a drastic drop in the incidence of the disease. (As with other vaccines, however, the one for measles has produced adverse reactions in some children.)

The characteristic bumpy, pinkish rash of measles appears on the face and neck about one to two weeks after exposure to someone with the disease. The rash is preceded by fever, coldlike symptoms, cough, and conjunctivitis, which may go largely unheeded until the rash itself appears, subsequently spreading over the body. The disease is contagious for about nine days, starting about four days before the telltale rash makes its first appearance; consequently, measles can be spread before the infected person knows the disease is present.

Rubella, or German measles. This disease is also characterized by a pimply, pink rash that begins on the face and then spreads down the body. The German measles rash takes two to three weeks to develop following exposure and is accompanied by lymph gland swelling on the back of the head and the neck.

German measles itself is a mild disease, but it is very dangerous for pregnant women. If a woman contracts rubella during her first three months of pregnancy, she is liable to suffer an abortion or stillbirth or to give birth to a child with physical defects and possible retardation. A rubella vaccine was introduced in 1969, and through a program of childhood vaccination it is hoped that girls will not be susceptible to the disease when they reach childbearing age.

Rabies. This infectious disease of mammals, and especially of carnivores, is caused by a virus that is often present in the saliva of infected animals. Animal bites are the main source of transmission of rabies to humans. The virus invades the central nervous system, producing numbness and tingling of the extremities, restlessness increasing to uncontrollable excitability, fever, paralysis, gagging, agitation, convulsions, muscle contractions, and respiratory paralysis that can lead to death. Very painful spasms of the muscles of the larynx and the throat make it impossible to drink water, which is why the disease is often called "hydrophobia."

Unless the victim receives immediate treatment following exposure, before symptoms begin to appear, the disease is likely to prove fatal. Antirabies treatments carry some risks in themselves, sometimes triggering an autoimmune reaction known as postvaccinal encephalitis. Before beginning the treatment, therefore, doctors try to locate the animal that administered the bite to determine whether it had rabies. If the animal cannot be found, the treatment is undertaken anyway, since the risk of treatment is much less than the near certainty of death from the disease itself.

Smallpox. Before this formerly dread disease was brought under control through vaccination, smallpox was infamous for being highly contagious. The disease typically began with a three-day period of headaches and backaches, followed by a skin eruption all over the body which often produced permanent pits and scars. Death often resulted from the toxins released by the virus or from the streptococcal bacteria that sometimes accompanied the disease.

Although the world is better off to be rid of smallpox, the vaccine is now known not to have been as harmless as was originally believed, and there is no reason to continue smallpox vaccinations today.

Mumps. Another viral disease that is now prevented through vaccination, mumps mainly affects the salivary glands. In severe cases, it may involve swelling of the pancreas and of the testicles. Among postpubertal males, about half the affected testicles become atrophic to some degree, but the disease rarely produces actual sterility. The incubation period of mumps is from two to three weeks, and the infected individual is contagious for as long as the salivary glands are swollen.

Hepatitis. There are two major forms of this potentially serious disease. Type A, previously known as "infectious hepatitis," is spread largely by fecal contamination. It can be contracted from eating infected shellfish or other contaminated food or drink, or by inhaling airborne virus from someone sick with the disease — often a family member. Type B is mainly transmitted by injection into the blood stream — through blood transfusions; the use of contaminated needles when taking drugs, getting tattoos, performing acupuncture, or piercing ears; or infected blood samples getting into open cuts or abrasions. Other methods of transfer, involving intimate contact such as oral sex or even the sharing of toilet articles, are also possible but much less likely.

Both types of hepatitis attack the liver. The symptoms include gradually increasing dizziness, which progresses to severe fatigue, loss of appetite with aversion to cigarettes, nausea, stomach pains, and liver swelling. The damage to the liver prevents that organ from performing its blood-cleaning function, and so toxins build up in the body, causing further damage.

Type A hepatitis does not last as long as Type B and is not generally as serious. Type A is characterized by elevated IgM levels. About three hundred thousand cases of Type A are reported each year in the United States.

Type B is more serious. Typically it is marked by the appearance of jaundice, a yellowing of the skin due to improper filtering of red blood cells and the accumulation of waste products in the blood stream. Other complications of hepatitis B can include cirrhosis of the liver and liver tumors. The liver damage is thought to be produced by the immune response to the hepatitis B virus antigens, and people with hepatitis B are believed to have a defect in their T suppressor cell production (Oda 1976).

In most cases, hepatitis clears up after four to eight weeks, but in many cases it leads to a subsequent impairment of immune functioning. This may be due to the heavy concentration of white cells needed in the liver, which reduces their numbers in other parts of the body. People who have had hepatitis B often develop other diseases later on.

Herpes. This illness has become all too familiar as one of the major viral diseases of the 1980s. It is ameliorated by high doses of antioxidants (vitamins A, C, E, and selenium) and to some extent, the amino acid lysine.

Antibiotics don't kill viruses! While we are on the subject of viruses, we should point out that antibiotics are *not* helpful in fighting viral infections. Antibiotics, such as tetracycline, sulfa drugs, penicillin, and many others, operate through various mechanisms to fight bacteria. Some also combat rickettsia (micro-organisms that have characteristics of both viruses and bacteria), fungi, and protozoa. But, because viruses live within the body's cells and depend on the host cell's metabolism for reproduction, the only way to combat viruses chemically is by attacking the cells that they infest. A few antiviral drugs do exist, but they have potentially damaging side effects because they are toxic to body cells.

Sometimes antibiotics are given in viral illnesses to prevent bacterial infection that may accompany the virus, as in the case of streptococcal infection accompanying smallpox. However, the overuse of antibiotics should definitely be avoided, since organisms that are resistant to the specific antibiotics used can multiply when competing micro-organisms are removed. For example, excessive use of antibiotics is considered one of the reasons why the yeast candida, which can become a fungus in the body, has become a major health problem, as will be discussed in Chapter 13.

Vitamin C fights viral diseases. As we have mentioned earlier, megadoses of vitamin C have been successfully utilized to destroy the viruses responsible for a full spectrum of serious illnesses.

While the case continues to be argued in medical circles, millions of people now take vitamin C at the first sign of a cold. Why some manage to eliminate symptoms rapidly while others report "no effect" may have more to do with dosage than previously believed. As we will discuss in Chapter 9, Robert Cathcart III, M.D., has treated more than twelve thousand patients for viral illnesses — ranging from the common cold to AIDS. His new method for determining vitamin C dosage, which he terms "bowel tolerance," was summarized in Chapter 6. Basically, Dr. Cathcart determines dosage on the principle that "the sicker you are, the more vitamin C you can take without developing diarrhea."

BACTERIA

Bacteria are one-celled organisms that are found throughout the body. As you know, some bacteria are quite beneficial. For example, certain bacteria that normally live in the intestines are responsible for manufacturing vitamin K, biotin, and other B vitamins that your body requires. When the normal balance of bacteria in the digestive tract is disturbed (for example, because of a reduction of fiber in your diet or when you take broad-spectrum antibiotics), other, harmful bacteria may take over. Bacteria do much of their damage through the production of toxins, rather than through the cell destruction characteristic of viral infestations.

Harmful anaerobic bacteria in the intestine produce toxins that are suspected of contributing to cancer of the colon. As another example, the bacteria responsible for botulism (a severe, often fatal form of food poisoning) produce the deadly botulin toxin, an extremely potent nerve poison.

One of the immune system's strategies against bacteria is to use antibodies to hinder the production of bacterial toxins. The antibodies attach to antigens at or near the point where the toxin is produced or released, physically blocking the exit of the toxins. Antibodies may also split bacteria open, killing them. (This process is known as *lysis.*) Complexes of bacteria and antibodies may also activate the system that produces local inflammation, raising the temperature in the area to a point that may be lethal to the invading bacteria.

When you develop a bacterial disease, it is because the pathogenic organisms have gotten past your humoral immunity defenses — the B cells and the antibodies they produce. (Viral infections, on the other hand, are largely the result of weakened T cell immunity.) Once you have survived an attack by a particular bacterium, you are usually safe from contracting that disease in the future, since your immune system "remembers" the specific pathogen, as we have described previously, and is able to produce antibody quickly to combat it.

Minerals can increase your risk of infection! While this book strongly recommends your using nutrition and supplements to stimulate immunity to disease, bear in mind that recent discoveries show that some nutrients once considered to be generally beneficial are *to be avoided* in certain cases.

You should discontinue your multivitamin pill when you have a bacterial infection because the zinc it contains, while "a potent stimulator of T helper-cell immunity and T cell-dependent humoral immunity" (Rosenbaum 1984), severely inhibits the phagocyte response so critical in killing harmful bacteria. Also, the iron contained in a multivitamin tablet actually stimulates the growth of bacteria (and viruses)! For details of these findings, please refer back to Chapter 6.

BACTERIAL DISEASES

With that warning regarding minerals, let us turn to an overview of a few bacterial illnesses.

Whooping cough. Whooping cough, or pertussis, is a highly contagious bacterial infection that specifically affects the epithelial tissues lining the lungs. Although it can occur at any age, about half of the cases develop before the age of two. For older children and adults (except debilitated elderly people), the disease is not usually serious, but it can be life threatening for very young children.

The most characteristic symptom of the disease is a deep paroxysmal or spasmodic cough, which usually ends in a high-pitched, prolonged whooping inspiration, for which the disorder is named. The cough is often accompanied by the expulsion of thick, stringy mucus.

Immunization against pertussis is routinely begun in infancy, as a part of the series of DPT (diphtheria, pertussis, and tetanus) vaccinations, which conclude with entry into kindergarten. This controversial vaccine is known to produce local reactions and fever and has sometimes been associated with convulsions and neurological problems. While the medical profession continues to defend the safety of pertussis vaccine, many parents are understandably concerned about reports of dangerous reactions. The current status of this debate is summarized at the end of this chapter.

Botulism. This severe form of food poisoning is caused by a bacterium. The symptoms are *not* due to the bacteria themselves, but to the potent toxin they produce, which is then eaten in food. This toxin attacks the central nervous system, resulting in paralysis and death by asphyxiation in extreme cases. It is so potent that just $1/100,000$ of a gram of botulin toxin can be fatal.

Tetanus. This bacterial disease derives its name from the condition of continuous muscle contraction, or tetany, which is its hallmark. The bacterium usually enters the body through an open wound, as from a puncture by a rusty object. Other common sources of infection are the use of contaminated needles or exposure through open burns.

The bacteria interfere with the ability of muscles to relax, and the muscles progressively tighten until the victim dies. Some of the first muscles involved are those of the jaw, which gives the disease its common name of *lockjaw*. Among certain African tribes, the natives knock out a few front teeth, so that if they should happen to contract lockjaw they can still be fed through a straw until the disease becomes terminal. At the terminal stage, the muscle contractions are so strong that the bones often cannot withstand the strain, and some victims die as a result of broken bones puncturing their internal organs.

This terrible disease is now prevented through vaccination; it is included in childhood DPT shots, and adequate protection must be maintained later in life.

Diphtheria. Diphtheria vaccine is the third component of the DPT shots given during childhood. The disease is characterized by headache, high fever, coughing, bloody nasal discharge, and a sore throat, with puslike secretions. The toxins produced by the diphtheria bacteria can damage cells and produce nerve paralysis and heart inflammation. Diphtheria antitoxin is given to patients who have developed symptoms, to reduce the damage done by the toxins.

Cholera. The bacteria responsible for cholera enter the small bowel and produce a toxin that causes the actual symptoms. Although cholera is relatively uncommon in the United States today, it is epidemic in areas of Asia and Africa, and Americans are required to be immunized against the disease before traveling in those areas. There have been seven major worldwide pandemics of cholera since 1817, with the seventh and most recent having only a modest impact on the Western Hemisphere.

The disease produces watery diarrhea and vomiting, leading to loss of fluids and important minerals, with resultant general fatigue and body aches. The disease is usually self-limited, with recovery within three to six days. In severe untreated cases, fatalities can exceed 50 percent, but are reduced to less than 1 percent when fluids and electrolytes are adequately replaced through intensive hospital care.

Tuberculosis. In the nineteenth century, this disease was known as "consumption." On the basis of tuberculin testing, it is known that some fifteen million Americans have live tuberculosis bacteria in their bodies, yet the disease is inactive in most. About thirty thousand people in this country develop active cases of tuberculosis each year, and of these cases perhaps three thousand are eventually fatal. Over the past thirty years, treatment with a combination of drugs has been effective in preventing the former ravages of this disease. Today, tuberculosis tends to be concentrated among inner-city dwellers, ethnic minorities, and recent immigrants from areas where the disease is still common. However, it can still occur anywhere; malnourished alcoholics, for example, are at high risk for developing the disease.

The symptoms of tuberculosis include dry cough, episodes of breathlessness, fever, night sweats, general fatigue, loss of appetite and weight, and coughing up blood. Tuberculosis may attack any bodily tissue, but the lungs are usually the hardest hit, with nodules, cavities, and scars developing, which are detectable on routine chest x ray.

THE VALUE OF FEVER

Before moving on to parasitic diseases, we would like to comment on a hallmark of many infectious diseases — fever, or a generalized elevation of body temperature. Fever is one of the body's natural defense mechanisms for fighting a widespread infection. Most micro-organisms are sensitive to heat, and so a rise in temperature may itself be enough to destroy the invaders. You may feel uncomfortable when you have a fever, but perhaps you can take satisfaction in knowing that the fever is even worse for the pathogen. If you take aspirin or other drugs to reduce a fever, you may actually be doing more harm than good, since you may be allowing the invaders to live and multiply in your body. It is a good idea to resist the impulse to take aspirin at the first sign of increased temperature; let the fever do its defensive work for you.

Of course, when a fever is dangerously high, you may need to use temperature-reducing drugs. In general, infants and young adults can tolerate higher fevers than older people. A fever of 104 degrees is not unusual for a child, but can be life threatening for a sixty-five-year-old. In any case, follow the advice of your doctor, who will be able to distinguish between a minor fever and a dangerous one.

Remember that your body needs larger than normal quantities of water and energy in order to generate a fever. That's why it is important for you to rest and to drink liquids when you are sick. Water helps to stabilize body temperature because of its ability to hold heat; if not enough fluids are present during a fever, your body will "burn itself up."

PARASITES

Whereas bacteria are classified as plants, the parasitic pathogens are members of the animal kingdom. For years it has been the common view that most parasites were "immune" to our immune defenses. Since parasites are often too large to be phagocytized and are seemingly unaffected by T cells and antibodies, parasitic diseases were rarely thought to be related to immune failure. But this viewpoint has recently undergone revision. Patients with suppressed immunity are now found to have "exacerbated or disseminated" parasitic infections, which leads parasitologists to believe the immune system *does* in fact play a vital role in protecting us against most parasites (Cox 1984). Further, these organisms can seriously lower resistance to other, nonparasitic diseases by directly depressing immunity.

How parasites avoid immune defenses. *Acquired* immunity is the way we generally resist parasites. But these clever invaders have "learned" how to actively by-pass the immune response. This evasion causes disease and seriously constrains the development of vaccines. For these reasons, it is worth looking at a few key "tricks" used by parasites and some of the diseases they cause. Parasites evade killing cells by:

- going around dissolving enzymes
- inactivating toxic oxygen
- entering disguised as a host antigen
- releasing enzymes that break white cells
- releasing T cell inhibitors.

To overcome these evasive techniques, parasitologists are experimenting with means of *stimulating macrophages,* in an attempt to shift "regulatory balance in favor of the host instead of the parasite" (Cox 1984). As we saw in the nutrition chapters earlier in this book, macrophage production can be depressed or enhanced by various nutrients. To protect against some parasitic illnesses, prevention is, as always, the best cure. Once infection has occurred, large doses of macrophage-stimulating vitamins and minerals should be taken — vitamin C, selenium, and zinc, as well as vitamin E, which protects macrophages from free radical damage.

(Once again, remember that excess iron *reduces* macrophage action and should be avoided when you are ill.)

PARASITIC DISEASES

Since parasitic diseases are related to immune suppression, and since some *can* be prevented or controlled to some degree through nutrient therapy, we will discuss a few representative examples.

Protozoal diseases. Protozoa are the simplest organisms in the animal kingdom. These one-celled organisms can range in size from submicroscopic to visible with the naked eye. The following are examples of protozoal illnesses.

Amebiasis is an infection of the colon caused by an amoeba that can be spread either directly from person to person or indirectly through food or water. Poor hygiene and intimate contact promote the spread of the amoeba. It is common in this country among male homosexuals and among some institutionalized groups. The symptoms are often relatively mild but may include intermittent diarrhea and constipation, flatulence, and cramping abdominal pain. The liver can become involved, developing abscesses.

Giardiasis is an infection of the small intestine caused by a protozoan. It not only spreads among people in close quarters in populated areas, but has also become of particular concern among lovers of the great outdoors. Formerly pure streams and lakes in the wilderness have become increasingly contaminated with this protozoan, not only through human contamination, but also because many wild animals carry it. The disease causes nausea, gas symptoms, abdominal cramps, and diarrhea. When the illness is severe, there may be significant weight loss owing to malabsorption.

Malaria is an infection caused by a protozoan that enters the body through a mosquito bite. The mosquito acquires the parasite by feeding on the blood of an infected person. Malaria is marked by alternating periods of severe fever and sweating, and chills. The drug quinine is used to reduce the symptoms.

Sleeping sickness, or *trypanosomiasis*, takes two forms. One is caused by the bite of the African tsetse fly, and the other, known as Chagas' disease, is transmitted by the bite of a particular bug, contaminated with the bug's feces. Sleeping sickness is characterized by severe lethargy; if the victim is left to his own devices, he may waste away.

Metazoan diseases. Technically speaking, a metazoan is any multicellular animal — in other words, any animal except a protozoan. Characteristic metazoan parasites are worms, which are able to enter the human or animal host through their own devices or through the intricacies of their reproductive cycle (Keeton 1980).

Although these relatively large parasites may not readily succumb to even the strongest immune defenses, they can definitely weaken our immunity and, therefore, we will review them briefly.

Tapeworms belong to a group known as flatworms. They usually enter the body through poorly cooked beef. The larvae are encased in the muscle tissue of infested cattle, and if the infested beef is consumed without being adequately cooked and chewed, the larvae may enter the human intestinal tract, where they attach to the intestinal walls and steal food from the host by consuming it before the intestine can absorb the nutrients. Tapeworm victims, therefore, have a voracious appetite and yet lose weight. To complete its life cycle, the tapeworm buds off parts of itself that contain eggs. These eggs are excreted with the host's feces. If plants are fertilized with these contaminated feces and a cow eats these plants, the larvae develop, burrow into the cow's muscles, and repeat the cycle.

Trichinosis is a parasitic disease with a very similar cycle, involving the roundworm *Trichinella spiralis.* Here the intermediate host is the pig, and the worms burrow directly into human muscles. The larvae do their greatest damage to humans while they are tunneling (perhaps half a billion at a time) from the digestive tract to the muscles. Symptoms of trichinosis include severe muscular pains, fever, anemia, weakness, and localized swelling. Death can result, and victims who do not die may suffer permanent muscle damage.

Other roundworm parasites of humans include *ascarid,* which is similar to the tapeworm in its life cycle and its way of infesting the body; *hookworms,* which burrow into the feet from the ground and cause very debilitating disease; *pinworms,* which enter the body when unclean fingers, contaminated by worm eggs, are put into the mouth; and *filaria* worms, which are spread by mosquito bites and which infect the lymphatic system, blocking the movement of fluids and resulting in such disorders as elephantiasis.

A flatworm with an extremely complex life cycle is the blood fluke, *schistosome,* which infests untold millions of people in many parts of the world. After the larvae of this organism leave their snail host, they enter humans directly through the skin and eat their way into a blood vessel, where they are transported to the heart, lungs, and intestines. Infested people may suffer serious complications, including cough, rash, body pains, dysentery, anemia, loss of strength, emaciation, and possibly death due to lowered resistance to other infectious diseases.

FUNGAL DISEASES

Fungal diseases are a world unto themselves. They may be due to poor T cell reaction in susceptible people. Since fungi are not highly antigenic, the white cells do not seem to have much effect against them.

A major fungal disease, which is reaching epidemic proportions in the United States, is candidiasis. This has become such a serious health problem that it will be discussed separately in a later chapter.

HOW HIGH THE PRICE OF VACCINATION?

Many of the bacterial and viral diseases we have discussed in this chapter have virtually been eliminated in this country during the present century. Widespread vaccination programs are usually given the credit for this achievement, although improved sanitation and, for many, a more adequate diet have certainly been important factors.

Now that the sharply reduced incidence of these diseases has decreased the possibility of infection, people are beginning to take a critical look at how safe these vaccines really are. It seems in some cases that the possible risks may outweigh the benefits of continued vaccination programs.

The potential dangers vary from one vaccine to another. At present, the pertussis component of childhood shots is the center of the greatest controversy. Some parents and physicians have even suggested that DPT shots may be causally linked with some cases diagnosed as "sudden infant death."

More children die *each year* from sudden infant death syndrome (SIDS) than the total number of all AIDS cases recorded since 1981, yet little research money has been allocated to study the possible relationship of some of these deaths to the DPT (diphtheria, pertussis, and tetanus) vaccine.

Before we look at a few concerned physicians' comments on the dangers of this vaccination, we must review how vaccination works and where the vaccine comes from.

How vaccination works. Vaccination, or immunization, is a method for artificially inducing immunity to a specific pathogenic disease. The recipient of the vaccination has not previously been exposed to the pathogen in question. The idea is to expose the individual to a weakened or dead strain of the disease organism so that the immune system can manufacture antibodies specific for its antigens. Later, if the individual does become exposed to the natural form of the pathogen, the immune system will "remember" the antigens, produce antibody, and prevent the harmful effects of the pathogen.

Since Jenner in 1796 first used cowpox vaccine, derived from cows, to protect humans against smallpox, medical research has developed a number of vaccines to protect us from various viruses, bacteria, and bacterial toxins. Today vaccines exist against the following diseases: cholera, diphtheria, influenza, measles, mumps, poliomyelitis, Rocky Mountain spotted fever, rubella, smallpox, tetanus, tuberculosis, yellow fever, and pertussis. Not all of these vaccines are guaranteed to completely prevent the respective diseases.

Today children are routinely vaccinated in infancy and again on entry into school. These vaccinations are credited with having virtually eradicated many diseases that were formerly massive killers of the young — but not without serious side effects in many children, as we will see below.

Immunizations are also required for many foreign travelers. Before going to another country, you may have to undergo immunizations for diseases that are common in the country you will be visiting.

Immunization may be considered either active or passive. In *active immunization,* a weakened or killed strain of the pathogen is injected directly into the person for whom it is intended. Active immunization may protect the recipient for a short time, or for life, or anywhere in between depending upon which pathogen is concerned. *Passive immunization* introduces the pathogen first into another organism, which manufactures specific antibodies. Then these antibodies are introduced into the final recipient. This procedure is called passive because the second recipient does not have to manufacture any antibody. Passive immunization generally results in an acquired resistance of shorter duration.

New doubts raised about vaccination. Despite the tremendous life-saving gains that have been attributed to massive public immunization programs, critics argue that some, if not all, vaccinations may presently do more harm than good. Because of the adverse reactions to some vaccines, people are questioning whether immunizations are necessary, especially in a population where the disease in question has been all but wiped out. For example, several European countries no longer require children to receive pertussis vaccine before entering school, owing to thousands of reports of shock, convulsions, and brain damage in vaccinated children. Similarly, the Centers for Disease Control (CDC) of the American Public Health Service have been urging doctors to abandon the practice of giving smallpox vaccinations as a matter of routine. In India homeopathic physicians trace many otherwise unexplainable maladies to the long-term aftereffects of smallpox vaccination.

Trouble with the DPT shots. All children in this country are routinely given immunization against diphtheria, pertussis, and tetanus and cannot enter school without it. But no injection of a foreign substance is without its price, and there is currently a lot of concern about the price of this one. As already mentioned, criticism focuses on the pertussis part of the vaccine.

According to Dr. Benjamin Nkowane of the Centers for Disease Control, of the eighteen million DPT injections given yearly (children receive a series of three), an estimated one in three hundred thousand causes permanent brain damage (McGrath 1984). Even this conservative estimate would yield sixty brain-damaged children a year.*

---

*An earlier study, known as the UCLA Study, published in 1980 shows one major seizure for each 875 children immunized! This represents a reaction rate more than ten times as great as the study generally cited by pediatricians.

Defending the shots, Dr. Martin Smith of the American Academy of Pediatrics is quoted as saying that one in every twelve thousand cases of whooping cough itself causes brain damage. The missing link in this argument is that it ignores the fact that many question the very ability of the vaccine to *prevent* pertussis reliably in the first place.

Made from the toxic bacteria that cause the disease, the pertussis vaccine is known to be an impure serum. Acknowledging this, Dr. Nkowane of CDC is quoted as follows:

> We do realize that this is not the best vaccine. No one knows what causes the brain damage and this is a crude vaccine. The vaccines for diphtheria and tetanus use only a specific portion of the bacteria, but the pertussis vaccine uses the whole bacteria. (McGrath 1984)

He also points out that no government studies are presently under way to assess the effects of DPT vaccine. The only major study of DPT's effects during the forty years the vaccine has been in use was conducted by the Food and Drug Administration and the University of California at Los Angeles in 1978. That study showed "a higher incidence of severe shock and other serious reactions than government figures indicate. According to the study, one of every 1,750 injections results in seizures or shock, but the research did not follow the affected children to see whether they sustained permanent damage" (McGrath 1984).

DPT suspected in sudden infant death. While the pediatrics Redbook, published by the American Academy of Pediatrics, does not mention SIDS among the possible severe side effects of DPT shots, the *Physicians' Desk Reference,* compiled by the drug manufacturers themselves, does say that the pertussis component of the DPT vaccine is "a possible link to SIDS."

A small newspaper in Contra Costa County, California, recently published a story that deserves national coverage (McGrath 1984). This story reports of a national parents' coalition calling for further study of the link between DPT and brain damage and of a correlation between the vaccine and crib death.

The situation is confused by tragedies in which SIDS seems to have been the wrong diagnosis. A Contra Costa County physician, Dr. Kevin C. Geraghty, researched several cases where DPT shots appeared to be connected to the sudden infant death syndrome. He reported:

> "We have talked to the families. These are not crib deaths where the child is found dead. . . . They are giving cat-like cries associated with encephalitis (inflammation of the brain). We talked to the parents of four SIDS children in Contra Costa who died within four days of receiving DPT. The kids were toxic, flaccid. Their brains are being blown out," said the pediatric immunologist and allergist. (McGrath 1984)

Where does this leave you as a parent? Should you vaccinate your child or not? The law in most states requires that you do. But you must be prepared to insist that your doctor listen very carefully to your family medical history, especially that of your child. Any previous signs of reactions to vaccinations, or any peculiar reaction by your baby to the first in the series of shots, is a strong reason to discontinue the series.

A homeopathic indictment of DPT. Besides brain damage and possible death, DPT injections can result in "a variety of other chronic complaints," according to another crusading physician, Richard Moskowitz, M.D. Dr. Moskowitz is a homeopathic physician with much direct experience treating children who have been injured by vaccines. In his practice, he has observed that vaccines produce a variety of symptoms of their own, sometimes much more serious than the original disease and almost always more difficult to recognize.

At a medical conference, he related several case histories to illustrate the dangers of vaccination. An eight-month-old girl had suffered bouts of fever, approximately one month apart. On investigation, these fever episodes were each found to have occurred after one of her series of DPT injections. Treatment with a homeopathic preparation* of DPT vaccine eliminated recurrences of the symptoms (Moskowitz 1984). Dr. Moskowitz writes:

> Since that time, I have seen at least half a dozen cases of children with recurrent fevers of unknown origin, associated with a variety

---

* Homeopathic remedies are extremely dilute preparations of the substance that in a healthy person would produce the symptoms from which the patient is suffering. For an overview of the homeopathic interpretation of vaccination and other illness, see Weiner and Goss.

of other chronic complaints, chiefly irritability, temper tantrums, and increased susceptibility to colds, tonsillitis, and ear infections, which are similarly traceable to the pertussis vaccine, and which responded successfully to treatment with the homeopathic DPT nosode. Indeed, I would have to say, on the basis of that experience, that the pertussis vaccine is probably one of the major causes of recurrent fevers of unknown origin in small children today. (Moskowitz 1984)

Dr. Moskowitz saw another infant who was showing blood abnormalities in the range of leukemia following a DPT shot. Later, when he saw a five-year-old with chronic lymphocytic leukemia, which also seemed to date from a DPT vaccination, he became even more concerned about the dangers of this routine medical procedure.

The idea that vaccinations might also be implicated in some cases of childhood leukemia was shocking enough in itself, but it also completed the line of reasoning opened up by the previous case, for leukemia is a cancerous process of the blood and the blood-forming organs, the liver, the spleen, the lymph nodes, and the bone marrow, which are also the basic anatomical units of the immune system. Insofar as the vaccines are capable of producing serious complications at all, the blood and the immune organs would certainly be the logical place to begin looking for them.

It was this case that convinced me, once and for all, of the serious need for public discussion of our collected experiences with vaccine-related illness, precisely because rigorous experimental proof will require years of investigation and a firm public commitment that has not even been made yet (Moskowitz 1984).

Lawsuits threaten supply of vaccine. Two major drug manufacturers (Wyeth and Connaught laboratories) stopped production of pertussis vaccine in 1984, rather than pay extraordinarily higher rates for liability insurance owing to its higher rate of side effects as compared with other vaccines.

This means, in practical terms, that the vaccine for each childhood disease is now made by a different manufacturer, and the old DPT vaccine is no longer available. So, parents now have the option of choosing to omit one or more of the "recommended" childhood vaccines. Until safer vaccines are developed, this is a wise decision.

However, children *are* required to have DPT shots as a condition of entry into public schools. Therefore, the question arises of who is responsible if the children suffer damage. Lawsuits against drug manufacturers may actually remove the pertussis vaccine from the market. A proposed U.S. Senate bill would compensate families of children damaged by DPT or other vaccines required by the government. This is small comfort to the parents of children who have already been injured.

The Japanese are testing a new serum that is supposed to be purer than the one in use in this country, but even if the Japanese vaccine does prove to be safer, it will be two to five years before it is available in the United States.

In the meantime, parents will have to grapple with this medicolegal dilemma. Religious or medical exemptions from compulsory vaccination are sometimes obtainable. For children with a history of suspected adverse reaction to a DPT or other shot, it would be advisable for their parents to confer with a pediatrician about obtaining exemption from further shots in the required series.

∘ 9 ∘

Cancer: The Immunity Connection

SIXTY TRILLION CELLS make up our body! What keeps them in harmony? How is the occasional "mad" cell, which wildly replicates itself, prevented from spreading the insurrection?

We are just beginning to "language" this process, and what we have learned is the result of studying how our immune system operates — more specifically, what happens when we encounter organ transplants, AIDS, and other shocks to our natural defenses.

What we are learning is that we can probably prevent many cancers and extend remission in others. Outright cure may even be possible, using conventional methods in combination with massive doses of certain nutrients and a complete health-revitalizing program.

Before getting into the details of some treatment regimens with exciting promise, we should again review immunity suppression and the outlines of this disease process.

WHAT SUPPRESSES IMMUNITY?

Immunosuppressive agents are factors that inhibit the efficacy of the immune response. You will remember that they may come either from outside or inside the body and that the individual may be exposed to them accidentally, or they may be given intentionally to suppress immune functioning or regulate other body functions.

Avoiding transplant rejection. As we discussed in Chapter 2, doctors sometimes find it necessary to use drugs to suppress the immune response so as to give a transplant a chance to become established. Currently a number of organs and tissues are being transplanted fairly routinely by doctors, including skin, bone marrow, kidneys, and corneas. Less common are transplants of the heart, lungs, liver, and pancreas.

Some transplants are being performed with a high degree of success. Cornea transplants, for example, are rarely rejected, partly because there is no shared blood supply between graft and recipient. In the case of skin grafts, the immune system will attack the graft unless the skin is taken from another part of the patient's own body.

Possibly you have been made aware of the problems of transplant rejection due to the publicity that surrounded the early heart transplant cases. Both the surgeons and the patients became international heroes, and the drama of threatened rejection episodes was followed closely on the news.

Although heart transplants have received the lion's share of the publicity, much of our present knowledge about transplant rejection was derived from tens of thousands of kidney transplant cases performed over a period of more than two decades. Of the more than thirteen hundred cases in 1972, for example, nearly half failed because of rejection (Strom 1982).

Transplant rejection may occur at various stages, with different parts of the immune system being involved. The first danger period is the minutes or hours immediately after surgery, when *hyperacute rejection* may occur. In the case of a kidney transplant, the kidney becomes soft, blue, and spotted, and the blood flow to the transplanted organ is drastically reduced. The kidney is completely destroyed within a few weeks. This type of rejection is caused by humoral antibodies. Between the first week and the fourth month after surgery, there may be *acute or intermediate rejection* — a cell-mediated reaction involving the natural killer cells. If the donor organ is transplanted from a cadaver, this type of rejection can take up to two years. *Late, or chronic, rejection* is generally seen in patients who have been undergoing prolonged drug therapy to suppress the immune system to prevent rejection. Another humoral antibody rejection, it takes the form of vascular occlusion, or blocking of the blood vessels (Hume 1971).

Whether a transplant is accepted or rejected is largely determined by a category of antigens called *histocompatibility antigens.* These antigens are genetically determined, and related people have fairly similar antigens. When a transplant is being considered, tissue typing can be done to determine how well matched the transplant donor and recipient are with regard to their histocompatibility antigens. In an organ transplant from one individual to another, the more closely related the two people are, the less likely it is that the recipient's immune system will reject the transplant. This is why blood relatives are the first choice as donors for procedures such as kidney transplants. People who receive a kidney transplant from a sibling or parent have an impressive 85 percent chance of surviving with the transplant for the rest of their lives (Hume 1971).

We will discuss specific immunosuppressive drugs in a later chapter. Here, we will examine a class of immunosuppressants that are virtually inescapable — the various forms of radiation in our environment.

Radiation. Radiation acts as an immunosuppressant by destroying the B cells, which are responsible for antibody production. The radiation source might be any high-energy electromagnetic radiation such as gamma rays, and the resulting degree of immune suppression depends on both the strength of the radiation and the total duration of exposure time. In order for radiation to destroy all of the antigen-sensitive cells in the body, the radiation would have to reach lethal or near-lethal levels and would destroy many other body cells as well, while possibly inducing mutations in the actively dividing cells.

While people are justly worried today about the consequences of nuclear warfare, there is also a just concern about exposure to so-called *low-level radiation,* which consists of the "background radiation" of natural radioactivity in the earth and cosmic rays, medical exposure to x rays and radioactive materials, and exposure to microwaves. While the dosage of radiation from medical sources is relatively small, it *is* larger than that received from background sources, and repeated x-ray exposure over our life span does not go away — it adds up.

Developing fetuses are most susceptible to damage from such

low-dose radiation, with many cases of juvenile cancer being traced to prenatal radiation exposure. In adults radiation seems to have the worst effect on the bone marrow, thyroid gland, lung, and female breast, with heavy exposure increasing the risk of cancer in these organs.

Sunlight and melanoma. Even sunlight — specifically, the ultraviolet (UV) radiation — can suppress the immune system. Excess UV exposure can result in skin problems including skin cancer, as well as in reduced immunological functioning. The use of some systemic medications (such as cortisone) can make the skin even *more* sensitive to the immunosuppressive effects of sunlight and increase the cancer risk (Harber and Baer 1978).

The threat of malignant melanoma is so great as to justify a few paragraphs about who is most likely to develop this disease and what precautions to take. (The source for the following discussion is Houghton and Viola 1981.)

Sunlight does not act *directly* as a carcinogen, but rather as a cancer "promoter," or "cocarcinogen." When sun exposure is added to heredity, hormones, damage to the skin, and chemicals in the air, you have increased cancer risk.

Where you take your sun is also significant. Melanoma rates rise, as might be expected, close to the equator. Obviously this is related to the increased intensity of the radiation (especially UV) at lower latitudes.

The parts of the body most often affected are those exposed during recreation; areas covered by bathing suits logically show fewer cases of cancer. According to the experts, "the highest concentration of melanomas occurs on the trunk, legs, and face, especially the lower legs of women and the trunk of men." Also as we would expect, the lighter the skin, the greater the number of cases.

Who is at risk?

> The classic phenotype of a person who develops melanoma is a blond or redhead with blue eyes, freckles, and fair skin; who tans poorly and sunburns easily (however, most persons who develop melanoma do not precisely fit this phenotype). (Houghton and Viola 1981)

As we would also expect, dark-skinned peoples have much lower melanoma incidences. Thus, blacks, Orientals, and Hispanics are generally safe from melanoma, with the exception of the feet and mucous membranes, which should be protected.

Queensland, Australia, offers the worst possible set of circumstances — the people are light skinned, and they live close to the equator. Unfortunately these people have the world's highest incidence of melanoma. As we would expect, the black-skinned aborigines rarely develop this disease.

Factors other than skin pigmentation and latitude of sun exposure may include sunspot cycles (UV radiation increases during periods of maximum sunspot numbers); a lessening of the protective effects of the earth's ozone layer due to atmospheric pollution, including the release of aerosols; time of day of exposure to the sun (the less intense the better); genetic susceptibility; additional immune suppression; hormones; and occupation.

Surprisingly, farmers, construction workers, and others in outdoor occupations have relatively *low* melanoma rates. This disease is more common among professionals and managerial people, leading to the conclusion that the occasional, intense exposure to sunlight by people with untanned skin, *not* chronic sun exposure, places us at the greater risk.

What can we do to protect ourselves? The obvious, common sense precautions are best: use a "sun-blocking" suntan lotion; expose yourself only *very gradually* to the sun (do not try to get a great tan on a weekend binge); and avoid midday exposure, when the sun is most intense.

Small dosages of sunlight stimulate the immune system (and help our bodies manufacture calciferol, or vitamin D), while great, intense exposure to the sun can actually suppress our immune function. This is another reason to think twice before joining the newly popular tanning parlors. The price of a "new skin" may be very high indeed.

Other immunosuppressants. Other agents that suppress immunity, as we have already seen, are cortisonelike steroids, cytotoxic chemicals, environmental pollutants such as pesticides and heavy metals, stress, malnutrition, microbes, alcohol and other drugs, and allergens.

Now that we have reviewed some of the immune suppressants and how they might relate to cancer, we should next look at the cancer process itself.

WHAT IS CANCER?

Thousands of books and hundreds of thousands of scientific articles have been written to answer this question. We can not do
more here than outline some of the leading theories of cause and
some of the more exciting avenues of cure.

We know that some of us are more susceptible to cancer than
other people. This is thought to be due to a genetic predisposition,
which means that if cancer "runs in your family," you especially
will want to avoid any contact with carcinogens or other im-
mune-depressing agents, while also *stimulating* your immune system.

When a genetically susceptible person is exposed to a cancer-
causing virus or repeated insults (smoking, air pollution, food additives, etc.), that person is particularly susceptible to the disease
because of a poor innate ability to defend against it.

WHAT KINDS OF CANCER ARE THERE?

There are more than a hundred different varieties of cancer, divided into four main categories — *sarcomas,* which affect muscle
and bone; *carcinomas,* which affect skin or organ linings; *leukemias,*
which are cancers of the blood; and *lymphomas,* which affect the
lymphatic system.

By its mere presence, a cancerous growth is not so deadly.
Rather, cancer kills through many different mechanisms. It may
weaken the body generally, cripple specific vital organs such as
the lungs, exert pressure on the brain, obstruct air or blood passageways, destroy blood coagulants leading to uncontrolled
bleeding, or block the immune system from performing its defensive work (Levitt et al. 1979).

NATURAL WEAPONS AGAINST CANCER

Your immune system, if it is functioning properly, is constantly
on the lookout for abnormal cells, and it has several different
weapons for battling cancer. Cytotoxins destroy dispersed cell
tumors and help to prevent metastasis (the spread of cancer from
one location to another) by locating and destroying small tumors

before they have a chance to grow. Some T cells are stimulated by tumor antigens to release *lymphokines* (defensive cells that are *not* antibodies), which call the macrophages into action. The resulting tissue damage may involve healthy cells as well as the cancer cells. Finally, natural killer cells may directly attack and destroy cancer cells with the help of IgG (Cunningham 1978).

Another naturally produced weapon against cancer cells is interferon. Produced by white blood cells when attacked by a foreign virus or cancer cells, human interferon is a protein that acts by arresting the replication of the threatening virus.

As mentioned in a previous chapter, interferon genes have been identified, removed from cells, and cloned in bacteria as well as in human cells. Highly purified interferon is being slowly produced in laboratories and should soon be available for use against cancer cells and other viral illnesses. Of course it will be expensive, and the most desirable alternative to laboratory-derived interferon is to discover how our body produces the substance, naturally, and stimulate this process.

What causes the body to produce interferon? Substances that act as antigens and stimulate T or B cells also stimulate interferon production. The trick is to stimulate a higher rate of interferon production without having to increase the load of antigen, or harmful substance. In experiments, many different kinds of substances have been found capable of inducing interferons. These interferon inducers include naturally produced toxins, cancer-causing chemicals, low molecular weight compounds, and double-stranded RNAs (ribonucleic acids, which are acids found in certain portions of cells and which play key roles in chemical reactions within cells). These RNAs are one of the most promising types of interferon inducers. They are the most effective, least toxic, and most broadly active of all inducers investigated. For this reason, special nucleic acids are being pursued as the greatest hope in naturally induced interferon. Much is known about the "ideal" nucleic acid, including its chemical structure and molecular weight, and we should soon see some breakthroughs in this important natural class of interferon inducer. While we wait for such breakthroughs, we will have to rely on the opinion of some doctors who believe that vitamin C may also stimulate interferons, naturally, within our body.

HOW CANCERS GET STARTED

Cancer has many ways of evading your immune defenses (Cunningham 1978). The immune system may be deficient in natural weapons. Such a deficiency may have been present since birth, or it may be a temporary problem caused by some other illness or by immunosuppressive agents. Another reason the cancer initially may be able to sneak through the defensive barriers is that it is very small; after all, cancer starts as only one cell. Later, once it has become established, the cancer may grow too fast to be eliminated. As we have learned, the immune system's "memory" operates by keeping small amounts of an antigen around as an aid to recognizing that antigen in the future. These small amounts do not trigger the immune response. Possibly, a small cancerous growth may similarly escape attention. The immune system may then develop tolerance for a cancerous growth that has been around for some time.

In addition, a tumor may actively defend itself against macrophages. It has been speculated that a tumor may be able to bury its surface antigens in the center of its mass of cells, where they are inaccessible to the attack of macrophages. Or, a tumor may be so similar to normal body tissues that it provokes only a weak immune response and is, therefore, difficult for the body to reject. The immune system also might be malfunctioning — either in general, or specifically in dealing with tumors. And, finally, the immune system becomes less efficient with age. If a tumor is patient enough, and nothing else kills a person first, the immune system may eventually break down, giving the tumor free rein to grow. The time in life when this breakdown occurs varies from one person to the next and seems to depend partly on genetics.

AVOIDING A SEA OF CARCINOGENS

We are continuously exposed to roaming cancer cells in our bodies and to agents that suppress our immunity. Some of us succumb, while others of us have a strong enough resistance (that is, immunity) and do not contract this disease.

In addition to the level of resistance to cancer (and other illnesses) that we inherit, we must learn to resist cancer by limiting our exposure to agents and situations that suppress our immune system. Study after study supports the relationship, for example, between occupational exposure to powerful carcinogens in certain industries and the number of people in those industries who develop cancer. Creosote, rubber, asbestos, tar, and other volatile compounds increase the risk of cancer, and workers in these industries have far higher rates of the disease than the population at large. Pesticides, drugs, tobacco, automobile exhaust, certain food additives, radiation, and other agents actively suppress our immunity and must be carefully avoided, as far as possible. Despite industrial public relations efforts that attempt to lull us into a false sense of security, we *do* live in a sea of carcinogens and can greatly limit our exposure to these immune suppressants by common sense measures.

There is no question that a high level of immunity is your best protection against cancer. In addition to avoiding carcinogens, you can also actively enhance or stimulate your natural immunity through proper use of the foods and supplements discussed in Chapters 5 and 6.

You now have a good idea of what runs down our resistance. What is more important is what we can do to *prevent* cancer.

RAISING YOUR IMMUNITY LEVEL: DO VITAMINS AND MINERALS WORK?

VITAMIN C

Robert Cathcart III, M.D., has treated more than twelve thousand patients with vitamin C, for a wide variety of viral illnesses. Having much direct clinical experience with this immunity-enhancing vitamin, he has developed a practical method of determining how much vitamin C you need. This may be useful in preventing cancer or extending remissions when taken as part of an overall immune-enhancing plan.

According to Dr. Cathcart, "the sicker you are, the more vitamin C you can take." When you are well, about one to four grams (1000 to 3000 milligrams) per day is considered an adequate *maintenance level* of this nutrient. Should you begin to get sick, due to an

inordinate stress or exposure to some other immune suppres-
sant(s), you can increase your vitamin C intake without developing gas or diarrhea. Dr. Cathcart has repeatedly demonstrated
that diarrhea is the sign of your *optimal dose*. At this point, you
should back off your vitamin C dose by about 10 percent and
maintain that level until you begin to feel better, at which time
you should begin gradually decreasing your intake to the maintenance level.

An intake of *other* immune-stimulating nutrients, especially
magnesium, as outlined in Chapter 6, will be required with these
increased dosages of vitamin C.

Using "bowel-tolerance" dosages of vitamin C to treat viral illnesses has led to the trial of this vitamin in treating cancer. The
debate as to the effectiveness of vitamin C in cancer rests on two
or three differences between proponents and detractors.

As we mentioned in Chapter 6, Drs. Ewan Cameron and Linus
Pauling conducted a major treatment study in Vale of Leven
Hospital, Loch Lomondside, Scotland. In that original work, it
was proven that patients treated with ascorbate (vitamin C) *"lived
on the average over four times as long* as the matched controls. . . ."
The amount taken was 10 grams per day, in one hundred patients
with "advanced cancer." There were also one thousand other patients (controls) who were given the same treatment except that
they did *not* receive vitamin C.

It is important to remember that one of the authors of this
study, Dr. Cameron, is a surgeon who has treated cancer patients
for more than thirty years, first by conventional methods alone
and later with vitamin C (Cameron and Pauling 1980).

The Mayo Clinic trials. The detractors of vitamin C claim to
have "duplicated" Cameron and Pauling's work, but without see-
ing any improvement in patients who took this vitamin. Unfortunately, and significantly, in this first Mayo Clinic trial, the
patients had all "received heavy doses of cytotoxic chemotherapy." It is well established that this type of chemotherapy damages the immune system and most likely interferes with the
effective action of vitamin C. Moreover, the Mayo Clinic researchers *knew* that Pauling and Cameron's patients had not had
such cytotoxic chemotherapy, but chose to ignore this important
factor. As reported by the vitamin C proponents: "The value of

vitamin C is much less for patients when immune systems have been damaged by chemotherapy than for those (as in the Vale of Leven study) who have not received chemotherapy" (Cameron and Pauling 1980).

Another clinical trial, in Japan, supported the results seen in Scotland. Survival times were much higher (483 days, average) among patients who took high doses of vitamin C (5 grams or more per day) than among those who took low doses (0–4 grams per day). The latter group survived, on average, less than 174 days (Morishige and Murata 1978).

In their most recent report on vitamin C and cancer, the Mayo Clinic people loudly proclaimed the ineffectiveness of ascorbate. Again, however, their study was seriously flawed (Moertel et al. 1985).

In an interview with Dr. Cameron, at the Linus Pauling Institute of Science and Medicine, we learned why this pioneering cancer surgeon was angered by the Mayo Clinic report as it appeared in the *New England Journal of Medicine* (January 17, 1985).

The article does read well on superficial examination. A more careful analysis shows two key deceptions, or errors.

First, the vitamin C was stopped at the first sign of progression of the illness, an average of ten weeks. In an illness that usually runs two years (colorectal cancer), two and one-half months on vitamin C is not a long enough time period to judge its merits. By comparison, in the study in Scotland, cancer patients were kept on ascorbate indefinitely!

Second, there seems *not* to have been any systematic attempt by the Mayo Clinic researchers to test patient compliance in taking the vitamin! We have no way to know if the patients were actually taking the vitamin C on a regular basis. Further, among the controls, the researchers found 500 milligrams of ascorbate in their urine per day. It is a well-established fact that you see vitamin C in urine only if you are taking vitamin C. So, contrary to the design of this study, some controls were also taking the vitamin (ingesting about 2 grams a day will yield about 500 milligrams in the urine).

These problems with the study refute not vitamin C's effectiveness against cancer, but the researchers' credibility.

How much should you take? As a means of stimulating your immunity, vitamin C is safe, inexpensive, and readily available in foods. Dr. Pauling calculates our average daily need at 10,000 milligrams per day (10 grams), while other proponents feel that 1–3 grams per day is a reasonable range for maintaining immunity, with more required at the signs of illness, exposure to immune depressants (each cigarette depletes about 25 milligrams of C), or increased emotional stress.

Are there any harmful effects from high doses of vitamin C? Diarrhea, a common complaint among people who take vitamin C in high doses, is not a side effect but a desirable endpoint! It serves as an indicator of an individual's effective dose. By reducing the amount you are taking at the point of diarrhea by about 10 percent, you should be able to get maximum immune enhancement without this problem.

Gastritis is another common complaint with vitamin C. It is true that a pre-existing ulcer will hurt when you take ascorbic acid. But a normal stomach will not be affected. To take the vitamin without experiencing pain, should you have stomach ulcers, the buffered form of sodium ascorbate is considered best.

Burning urination has been reported, but in the experience of Dr. Cathcart — who has more clinical experience with this vitamin than any other physician — he has seen this complaint in only about one out of three thousand patients!

Another reported problem with vitamin C is that people become adapted or addicted to a high dose, and they may develop scurvy when they try to eliminate the vitamin. The point to remember here is to withdraw to a maintenance level after the high doses used during an acute illness. The trouble occurs when people eliminate the vitamin entirely; so total withdrawal is never recommended.

As for kidney stones, another reported side effect of high doses, clinical studies have refuted this claim — which originated as the result of *theory*. The theory was based on the assumption that some part of the breakdown products of ascorbate is oxalate, an acid that might bind with calcium to form calcium oxalate kidney stones. But, as a matter of fact, this does not happen.

Table 9 shows some fruits and vegetables and their vitamin C content.

TABLE 9

Selected Sources of Vitamin C

Food	Portion Size	Amount in Milligrams
Orange juice, freshly squeezed	1 cup	124
Orange juice, frozen, made from concentrate	1 cup	117
Green peppers, raw, chopped	½ cup	96
Grapefruit juice	1 cup	93
Papaya	½	85
Brussels sprouts, cooked	4 sprouts	73
Broccoli, raw, chopped	½ cup	70
Orange	1 medium size	66
Turnip greens	½ cup	50
Cantaloupe, fresh	¼ medium size	45
Cauliflower, raw, chopped	½ cup	45
Strawberries, fresh	½ cup	44
Tomato juice	1 cup	39
Grapefruit	½	37
Potato, baked	1 medium size	31
Tomato, raw	1 medium size	28
Cabbage, raw, chopped	½ cup	21
Blackberries, fresh	½ cup	15
Spinach, raw, chopped	½ cup	14
Blueberries, fresh	½ cup	10
Cherries, sweet, fresh	½ cup	8
Mung bean sprouts	¼ cup	5

Source: USDA Handbook No. 8

VITAMIN A

Less controversial as to its effectiveness in both preventing and treating cancer is the fat-soluble nutrient vitamin A. Like vitamin C, it can not be made in the body and must be taken in food as either vitamin A alcohol (known as retinol) and its chemical attachments (esters), or as beta-carotene (a provitamin that is split in the intestine into vitamin A).

In addition to its many other functions (outlined in Chapter 6), this vitamin plays a key role in oncology (Bollag 1983).

Since the 1920s, it has been known that a deficiency of vitamin A leads to the first step on the road to cancerous tissue, particularly in the lining of the respiratory, gastrointestinal, and genitourinary tracts.

Numerous studies in animals showed a beneficial effect of this vitamin. It prevented the appearance of squamous cell tumors in hamsters subjected to toxic levels of benzopyrene, a potent and volatile carcinogen (Bollag 1983).

Small epidemiological studies in humans also show the value of vitamin A, with a lowered cancer incidence related to levels of this vitamin found in the blood (Peto et al. 1981).

In another study, of sixteen thousand men, low levels of vitamin A (retinol) were clearly "associated with an increased risk of cancer," independent of age and smoking habits. The authors concluded that "measures taken to increase serum-retinol levels in man may lead to a reduction in cancer risk" (Wald, Idle, and Boreham 1980).

Another large study, this time of 1,954 middle-age men, led investigators to conclude that "intake of dietary provitamin A (carotene) was inversely related to the 19-year incidence of lung cancer. ..." In other words, those who took vitamin A through foods or supplements had greater protection against cancer than those who did not. Similar epidemiological studies in Norway and Japan, and case-control studies in Singapore, the U.S.A., and the United Kingdom show the same benefits of this vitamin, as reported in *The Lancet* for November 28, 1981 (Shekelle 1981).

In clinical studies, *retinoids* (a form of vitamin A) were shown to prevent the recurrence of bladder tumors, cause the regression of bronchial precancer in heavy smokers, and bring about regression of cancers in other tissues. The only caution was the potential side effects, which limit the usefulness of the retinoids (Bollag 1983).

How to take vitamin A. Because of the potential toxicity of large amounts of preformed vitamin A, we recommend that you take the beta-carotene form, as found in foods. Beta-carotene is converted in the body into vitamin A, but large amounts of it are not known to be toxic. It can lead to a yellowing of the skin, but this is reversible after excessive beta-carotene intake is stopped.

Large amounts are *not* recommended, however, and one or two

TABLE 10

Carotene Content of Common Foods

Food	Serving	Carotene (IU)
Papaya	½ medium size	8867
Sweet potato	½ cup, cooked	8500
Collard greens	½ cup, cooked	7917
Carrots	½ cup, cooked	7250
Chard	½ cup, cooked	6042
Beet greens	½ cup, cooked	6042
Spinach	½ cup, cooked	6000
Cantaloupe	¼ medium size	5667
Broccoli	½ cup, cooked	3229
Squash, butternut	½ cup, cooked	1333
Watermelon	1 cup	1173
Peaches	1 large	1042
Squash, yellow	½ cup, cooked	900
Apricots	1 medium size	892
Squash, hubbard	½ cup, cooked	667
Squash, zucchini	½ cup, cooked	600
Prunes	½ cup, cooked	417
Squash, acorn	½ cooked	234

Note: The values shown are for representative samples of the foods listed. Values for any specific sample will vary depending on where, when, and how it was grown and processed. Also, the proportion of beta-carotene in the food that is actually taken up by the body will vary depending on the person's nutritional state, the foods with which it is eaten, and other factors. In order to obtain beta-carotene content of foods in terms of retinol equivalents, divide the value in IU by ten.

Source: Bauernfiend, 1981

servings of beta-carotene-rich foods each day should offer adequate protection. (See Table 10.)

SELENIUM

Selenium, a trace mineral, is protective because it enhances immune functions when taken in moderate amounts. This mineral has been discussed in an earlier nutrition chapter, and here will only be reinforced in its relationship to cancer.

J. S. Prasad, M.D., Ph.D., and others have looked at the relationship between cancer deaths and dietary selenium intake in twenty-seven countries. Included in the study were different types of cancer, such as breast, lung, prostate, and ovarian. The results show that the higher the intake of selenium (up to a point), the fewer the cancer deaths (Prasad 1978).

R. J. Shamberger, Ph.D., and D. V. C. Frost, Ph.D., have looked at selenium intake and cancer, mainly in the United States. They reported that the higher the soil or crop level of selenium, the lower the cancer death rate (Shamberger and Frost 1969).

But the best evidence that selenium may prevent cancer comes from case-control studies. In patients with skin cancer, the level of this trace mineral in the blood was significantly lower than in 108 control subjects without cancer. That is, healthy individuals (without cancer) had *more* selenium in their circulation than did cancer patients (Clark et al. 1984).

Remember, selenium can be toxic above about 800 micrograms per day. The average American diet supplies between 50 and 160 micrograms, depending on where you live and in which soil your food is grown. Since most of us do not live in the parts of the Midwest and Southwest where soil selenium levels are high, it may be advisable to supplement with low amounts of this valuable trace mineral.

Amounts of selenium in foods are related to the food's protein content. Foods low in protein (such as fruits) contain little of this element. One last note: cooking does *not* cause large losses of selenium from most foods, but the dry heating of cereals causes up to a 23 percent loss (Prasad 1978).

Having seen which nutrients protect us against cancer, we now have to face one of the biggest "question marks" — whether this disease is communicable. It is worth looking at the practical implications of this provocative question.

IS CANCER COMMUNICABLE?*

Cancer in married couples. (Enck 1979)

Identical cancer in husband and wife. (Russ and Scanlon 1980)

---

*The title, structure, and quotes in this subsection are derived from Henry T. Lynch et al. at the Creighton University School of Medicine, Omaha, Nebraska (see Lynch, Schuelke, and O'Hara 1984).

Correlation between cancers of the uterine cervix and penis in China. (Li et al. 1982)

Immunodeficiency among female sexual partners of males with . . . AIDS. (Harris et al. 1983)

Multiple myeloma: houses and spouses. (Kyle and Greipp 1983)

Leukemia and lymphoma patients linked by prior social contact. (Schimpff et al. 1976)

These are the titles of scientific articles as they appear in the medical literature. Cancer's communicability is becoming a topic of concern as the incidence of AIDS (including Kaposi's sarcoma) continues to increase and our knowledge of the mechanism of transfer becomes more clear.

But as some researchers begin to ask if patients diagnosed as having AIDS should be quarantined to prevent the spread of this disease, another question arises: what about cancer patients in general?

If there is a viral agent involved in some cancers,[†] as we have good reason to believe, should we not consider quarantine as a reasonable procedure for patients diagnosed as suffering from such viral-related cancers?

This question has important sociological implications. But, before giving in to panic, it is reasonable first to look at the evidence implicating a "communicable agent." Then we can apply the immune-enhancing procedures outlined in this book to lessen our risk should we directly or indirectly contact a person suffering from this dreaded illness.

All people do not have equal cancer risk. "In the 'eyes' of a putative carcinogenic agent(s), all men are not equal in their susceptibility to the development of cancer" (Lynch, Schuelke, and O'Hara 1984). Both "nature" and "nurture" influence the degree of susceptibility.

Nature. Genetic susceptibility must not be overlooked in our analysis of the relative communicability of cancer. Several types of the disease have been clearly related to a hereditary factor.

[†]As we pointed out in an earlier chapter, many cancers are distinctly related to environmental insults (including nutritional negligence), which may allow the final causative organism — in this case a virus — to multiply.

Nurture. On the other side of the spectrum, we see a great many environmentally influenced cancers. Extreme examples include the nineteenth-century observations of very large numbers of cases of scrotal cancers among chimney sweeps; urinary bladder cancer related to benzopyrenes — especially from charcoal-broiled foods, but also from teas and coffees, and even more so from cigarettes, home heating, engine and industrial exhausts, etc. — and the eighty times greater cancer risk among asbestos workers who smoke, as compared to their nonsmoking fellow workers! These environmental factors raise cancer risk and, in the genetically susceptible, increase the possibility of communicability.

Another example of how environmental factors influence the development of cancer is seen in Nassau County, New York. Here, women have the trauma of a breast cancer rate 7.5 percent above the national average and 12 percent above the state rate for this disease. While the public health sages are studying the issue, women in this county may not know that they can take positive steps to reduce their risk for developing this disease, *now*. Ground water has been contaminated on Long Island for many years. Toxic materials were carelessly dumped without concern and have appeared in trace amounts for at least three decades. This is one critical factor. Another can be found in the types of diets of too many women in Nassau County. Two major ethnic groups, Jewish and Italian, appear in Nassau. The diets of these cultures are horribly high in fat and sugar while containing very little fiber, *a protective* nutrient. Looking at a nation with the world's *lowest* rate of breast cancer, Japan, we see women consuming foods that are very low in animal fats. Consisting mainly of fish, vegetables, and rice, this immune-enhancing diet would greatly protect against breast and other cancers, as has been concluded from numerous epidemiological studies. This is another area where politics, not science, dictates confusion. By controlling these two environmental factors (ground water and diet) the women of Nassau County, Long Island, and the United States could protect themselves from this dread disease.

Animal cancers related to viruses. "Given knowledge of evolutionary principles, it would appear unlikely that man would prove to be an exception to viral induction of cancer" (Lynch, Schuelke, and O'Hara 1984). Appendix 5 lists viruses known to be responsible for inducing cancer in various animals. The genetic susceptibility of the animal is known to be a crucial factor as to whether or not cancer develops. The point of this list is to demonstrate that viruses, which *are* communicable, in concert with other environmental factors do interact with susceptible genotypes and go on to develop into various kinds of cancer in animals. Man's animal heritage tends to make him likely to follow this pattern.

What we can do to reduce cancer's communicability. The evolving model regarding the genesis and evolution of cancer and other immunologic-related diseases consists of an *immune-compromised* person confronting a *causative organism* or series of organisms.

Without suppression of immunity, the mere association with the "causative" virus, protozoan, or other microbe will not be sufficient for the initiation of a cancerous process.

The most essential idea, then, is to *maintain immune readiness,* particularly if you are taking care of a person with cancer or another immune-related disease.

Malnutrition, inadequate intake of protective foods and nutrients, radiation, unending emotional stress, chemical and drug overload, and other events or agents known to breach the body's "defense department" are potentially deadly — especially when combined with exposure to a deadly virus, for example.

For a quick check of your relative immune status, you may want to return to Chapter 1 and the Im.Q. test. If your score is low and you are in contact with a seriously ill person on a regular basis, or have reason to believe you may have been exposed to a potentially deadly illness, it would be wise to see your physician and ask him or her to order a T cell evaluation and other appropriate measures of your immune function.

By following the resultant medical advice, in association with the immune-enhancing measures discussed throughout this book, you should see significant improvement in your T cell ratio and other indicators of immunity and be confident that you are doing what is reasonable to achieve maximum immunity.

○ 10 ○

Reducing the
Risk of AIDS

WHAT IS AIDS?

AIDS is an epidemic unlike any other. Those in the highest risk group and those for whom the bell tolls are also among our most politically active and astute groups as well.

Never before has an epidemic been viewed through such political lenses. When society as a whole has been at equal risk of infection, society as a whole has accepted the burden necessary for checking disease spread. AIDS, being highly *restricted* in its populations at risk (and a *difficult* disease to spread), presents an especially easy audience for control, as well as for eventual treatment. But politics now dictates where medical reason ought to prevail.

For five years the research establishment, in passive connivance with the homosexual lobby, has allowed us to fear that this disease was rapidly spreading into the general population. Led to believe that we were all *equally* at risk, we were subtly encouraged not to point the finger of blame at the specific group or groups we thought were the loci of infection. This strategy was meant to prevent stigmatizing homosexuals and drug addicts for infecting all of us, while also stampeding us into pouring a ransom of funds into studying AIDS, at the risk of neglecting other epidemics, notably childhood leukemia (children do not vote).

Now that panic is upon us and people are about to explode and demand common sense public health measures to control this epidemic, we are suddenly comforted by yet another Center for Disease Control (CDC) "expert" who tells us *not* to worry, that the disease is *not* spreading from the original groups at risk into the general population.

How can this be? Which position is true? Is this a universally communicable disease? To answer this question we must first seek an overview, returning later to "the politics of AIDS."

The complete destruction of the immune system and the development of any one of about twenty fatal diseases — including a form of cancer, a deadly pneumonia, as well as other killing fungal, bacterial, and viral illnesses — is a condition known as Acquired Immune Deficiency Syndrome, or AIDS.

In San Francisco, within a two-month period in 1985, first a nun and then an eighty-year-old matriarch died from a disease brought about by a blood transfusion taken from a person with AIDS, which had not yet been diagnosed. While this problem with contaminated blood may have been solved with the recent test for the presence of antibodies to the AIDS virus, the disease continues to spread.

We can greatly reduce, if not completely eliminate, our risk of developing this illness by first understanding the known and likely causes, and then by taking *preventive* steps.

There are clear links between the immune system and this disease. Therefore, without making this disease the entire focus of the "immunity" story, we have decided to limit our coverage of AIDS to this chapter, but in some detail. AIDS is a key window on the immune system. By applying what is being discovered about this disease and its transmission, as well as how it is being reversed by two alternative treatment programs, we can apply this knowledge to other diseases of immune failure.

To fully understand how we can reduce our risk of contacting or developing this disease, we should first familiarize ourselves with the problem as a whole.

BACKGROUND

Figure 4 shows the rising incidence of AIDS. It is alarming to see that of the ten thousand cases reported since 1981 more than *half* were reported in just ten months following June 1984!

Homosexual or bisexual men are still at highest risk (about 72

FIGURE 4

The Rising AIDS Epidemic

Acquired immunodeficiency syndrome cases and known deaths, by 6-month period of report — United States, 1981–April 1985

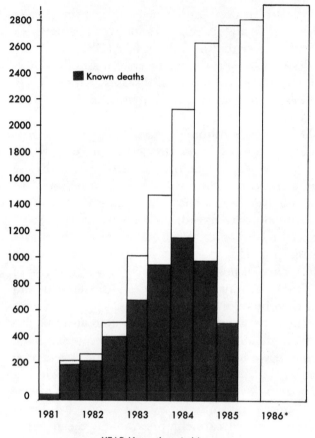

*Data incomplete and projected

Source: CDC, 1985b

percent of all cases in the United States), and intravenous drug users the next-highest risk group (about 17 percent). Table 11 shows a breakdown of adult AIDS patients in six groups, as well as gives statistics for children with the disease.

There are regional variations in this disease, not yet published. In San Francisco, most AIDS patients are homosexual men, while

TABLE II

AIDS in the U.S.

Acquired immunodeficiency syndrome (AIDS) patients, by patient group and date of report — United States, through April 1985*

Patient group	Before May 1983 No.	(%)	May 1983– April 1984 No.	(%)	May 1984– April 1985 No.	(%)	Total	(%)
Adult								
Homosexual/bisexual	992	(71.5)	2,070	(72.5)	4,199	(74.4)	7,261	(73.4)
IV drug user	233	(16.8)	510	(17.9)	942	(16.7)	1,685	(17.0)
Hemophilia patient	11	(0.8)	17	(0.6)	37	(0.7)	65	(0.7)
Heterosexual contact	13	(0.9)	23	(0.8)	45	(0.8)	81	(0.8)
Transfusion recipient	12	(0.9)	34	(1.2)	88	(1.6)	134	(1.4)
Other/unknown	126	(9.1)	202	(7.1)	333	(5.9)	661	(6.7)
Total	1,387	(100.0)	2,856	(100.0)	5,644	(100.0)	9,887	(100.0)
Pediatric								
Parent with AIDS or at increased risk for AIDS	11	(57.9)	27	(67.5)	43	(79.6)	81	(71.7)
Hemophilia patient	2	(10.5)	1	(2.5)	3	(5.6)	6	(5.3)
Transfusion recipient	2	(10.5)	8	(20.0)	5	(9.3)	15	(13.3)
Other/unknown	4	(21.1)	4	(10.0)	3	(5.6)	11	(9.7)
Total	19	(100.0)	40	(100.0)	54	(100.0)	113	(100.0)
TOTAL	1,406	(100.0)	2,896	(100.0)	5,698	(100.0)	10,000	(100.0)†

* An additional 3,402 cases were reported between May and September of 1985.
† By the end of 1986 there may be nearly 30,000 cases if present trends continue.

Source: CDC, 1985b

in New York, the incidence of the disease among IV drug users is much higher. Of the forty known heterosexual men in New York with the disease, all seem to have been infected by intimate association with high-risk individuals, namely female prostitutes who were drug users or in contact with AIDS patients.

There is no longer any doubt. This disease is sexually transmitted or passed through contact with infected blood. It is clearly *not* casually transmitted and more will be said about this issue later in the chapter.

It is important to know that of the 186 children with this disease as of late 1985, 72 percent came from families where one or both parents had AIDS or were at high risk for developing AIDS, 13 percent of the children had been given blood transfusions before they became ill, and 5 percent had hemophilia. Information on the parents of the remaining cases (10 percent) is incomplete. With these facts in mind, parents should not fear that this terrible disease is spreading without reasonable grounds for control. Blood for transfusions should be acquired from relatives and friends in sound health. (The new test for antibodies to the suspected AIDS virus is not perfect, which means blood supplies from general sources are of unknown safety.) The strong association between most children with AIDS and their relationship with infected individuals or blood products is further evidence that the disease is *not* casually transmitted.

The epidemiology of AIDS. AIDS was first diagnosed as an epidemic in 1981 and has since been found mainly in people from the various groups listed in Table 11. Up until 1984, Haitians were considered a group at high risk. It is significant that many Haitian people participate in rituals where scarification of the skin takes place. A transfer of blood from one person to another is a common part of these rituals, which may explain why such a great number of AIDS patients are Haitian. Further, detailed analysis of Haitian AIDS patients disclosed that most of them were either homosexual, bisexual, or IV drug users. Their being Haitian was not a risk factor unto itself.

Of course, the vast majority of all AIDS patients are homosexual or bisexual men, followed by intravenous drug users and hemophiliacs, and next by "heterosexual contacts" (that is, heterosexuals who were IV drug users or in intimate contact with AIDS patients), transfusion recipients, and last, others of unknown association.

AIDS IN EUROPE

As of December 31, 1984, 762 cases of AIDS had been reported from Europe. This also represents an alarming increase, from 235 cases reported in 1983 to more than 417 cases in 1984 (CDC 1985).

The highest rates of AIDS cases per capita were seen in Belgium and Denmark. Table 12 lists AIDS cases and rates in seven-

TABLE 12

AIDS in Europe: Overview

Reported acquired immunodeficiency syndrome cases and estimated rates per million population — 17 European countries*

Country	Oct. 1983†	July 1984	Oct. 1984	Dec. 1984	Rates‡
Austria	7	0	0	13	1.7
Belgium	38	0	0	65	6.6
Czechoslovakia	0	0	0	0	0.0
Denmark	13	28	31	34	6.6
Finland	0	0	4	5	1.0
France	94	180	221	260	4.8
Federal Republic of Germany	42	79	110	135	2.2
Greece	0	2	2	6	0.6
Iceland	0	0	0	0	0.0
Italy	3	8	10	14	0.3
Netherlands	12	21	26	42	2.9
Norway	0	0	4	5	1.2
Poland	0	0	0	0	0.0
Spain	6	14	18	18	0.5
Sweden	4	7	12	16	1.9
Switzerland	17	28	33	41	6.3
United Kingdom	24	54	88	108	1.9
Total	**260**	**421**	**559**	**762**	**2.0**

* Austria, Belgium, Czechoslovakia, Denmark, Finland, France, Federal Republic of Germany, Greece, Iceland, Italy, Netherlands, Norway, Poland, Spain, Sweden, Switzerland, and United Kingdom.

† These data were reported at the first European Meeting on AIDS held in Aarhus, Denmark, October 1983.

‡ Based on 1983 populations, INED, Paris.

Source: CDC, 1985a

teen European countries. It is important to note that 83 percent of the Belgian patients were Africans, of whom only eighteen lived in Belgium before the onset of the initial symptoms. In Denmark, *no* African or Caribbean patients have been registered with the disease. This difference is not yet understood.

As in the United States, the vast majority of cases are men (92 percent), mainly homosexual/bisexual (CDC 1985a). In Table 13, another peculiar statistic is displayed, the fact that 160 cases of the reported total of 762 cases occur among people with "no known risk factor." This high figure tends to frighten people into believing that the disease is spreading into the general population, without any known "reason." It is important to recognize that a person diagnosed as having AIDS may not want to divulge his or her activities with regard to sexual preference, frequency of contact, or use of intravenous drugs. Until we have a perfect method for assuring the validity of a patient's history, which is unlikely, we must assume that this disease is following *predictable* patterns of spread and that it does *not represent a threat to people in none of the known risk groups.*

This is not to minimize the terrible tragedy of the disease or the suffering of the patients. We must continue to seek an understanding of the causative organism(s), educate people as to eliminating risk factors, assure ourselves a "clean" blood supply, and evaluate all treatments that are reportedly successful in bringing about remission. A recent study by epidemiologists at the CDC estimates that more than four hundred thousand people may have been exposed to the suspected AIDS virus. The expected exponential increase in the number of cases in the near future emphasizes the critical importance in evaluating methods for stimulating the immune system to prevent the disease, as well as for treating the disease, should it be diagnosed.

WHAT CAUSES AIDS?

The suspected causative agent for AIDS appears to be *transmitted* in very much the same manner as hepatitis B, through contact with either blood or semen of the affected individual. Such contact can theoretically include *nonsexual contact* of mucosal surfaces (mouth, nose, rectum, genitals); contact with any open cut or sore; contact with any bodily secretions that subsequently enter through a skin abrasion; or contact with a mucosal surface. Currently there is no evidence that AIDS can be spread through the air — *it requires direct, moist contact.*

Acquired Immune Deficiency Syndrome is the ultimate breakdown of the immune system. For some still unknown reason(s), a

TABLE 13

AIDS in Europe:
Risk Groups and Geographic Origin

Acquired immunodeficiency syndrome cases, by patient risk group and geographic origin — 17 European countries, through December 31, 1984

Patient risk groups		European	Caribbean	African	Others	Total
			Nationality			
1.	Male homosexual or bisexual	514	2	5	16	537
2.	Intravenous-drug abuser	11	0	0	0	11
3.	Hemophilia patient	20	0	0	0	20
4.	Transfusion recipient (without other risk factors)	4	0	4	0	8
5.	1- and 2-associated	9	0	0	2	11
6.	No known risk factor					
	male	29	17	64	2	112
	female	15	4	29	0	48
7.	Unknown	3	1	9	2	15
Total		**605**	**24**	**111**	**22**	**762**

Source: CDC, 1985a

suspected infectious agent, likely the HTLV-III virus,* is able to strip the human body of its department of defense. How it does so is unknown, but the results are devastating. The suspected virus destroys healthy T helper cells.

There are contrasting theories of how this occurs. One theory is that a particular infectious agent is solely responsible for AIDS. Another theory maintains that AIDS is a result of the immune system being overloaded by numerous assaults from a wide variety of infectious and antigenic agents, as well as environmental pollutants. Other theories combine these two contrasting points of view.

Regardless of which theory is correct, the effect is the same —

---

*HTLV-III (Human T-lymphotropic virus, type III), LAV (Lymphadenopathy-associated virus), and ARV (AIDS-related virus) are each suspected to be the virus in question. We use only the HTLV-III initials in this chapter because all three "suspects" may eventually prove to be the same class of disease organism.

there is a gradual deterioration of immune function over a period of time. There is no one particular physiological marker to announce that AIDS has arrived. However, a lower T helper to T suppressor ratio (remember, the norm is about 1.8 helpers to 1 suppressor cell) may indicate immune deficiency and should be corrected at once using the nutrients and techniques outlined in this book.

Statistical links have been established between the frequency of certain viruses and the appearance of AIDS. However, correlation does not necessarily imply that the virus is a causative agent — it may just be along for the ride in an already immune-compromised host.

Evidence of the human T cell leukemia virus (HTLV-III) has been found in the blood of about one-third of the AIDS victims tested. HTLV-III is found in less than 5 percent of people without AIDS. Twelve percent of 172 non-AIDS hemophiliacs tested at the Harvard School of Public Health showed evidence that they had come in contact with HTLV-III, but that their immune systems were able to fight off the infection.

Another virus — cytomegalovirus (CMV) — is almost universal among AIDS patients. This virus is associated with a disorder known as Kaposi's sarcoma in Africans. However, the course of Kaposi's sarcoma in Africa differs considerably from its rapidly progressive course among United States AIDS victims.

Kaposi's sarcoma, or KS, appears in two very different forms. In the classic, or "background," form of the disease, first described in 1872, patients have normal T helper/suppressor ratios and generally lack the antibody to the HTLV-III virus (thought to be the "AIDS virus"). In the second type of the disease, which occurs mainly among AIDS patients who are homosexuals, a large percentage show suppressed T cell ratios.

The Epstein-Barr virus, associated with a type of cancer (Burkitt's lymphoma), is also frequent in people with AIDS. However, presence of a virus does not imply that the virus causes AIDS; it may be a secondary symptom.

Whatever the school of thought, all agree that AIDS is a disease of *immune regulatory failure*. Further, it is generally accepted that no *known* microbe can bring about AIDS by itself. A new microbe could bring on AIDS in an immune-suppressed person (Sonnabend and Saadoun 1984).

Precisely *how* this disease is initiated and progresses is the subject of much theorizing, all related to the immune system.

One disease model combines a known high-risk group (homosexual men) with environmental factors. These factors include:

- exposure and reexposure to many semens, which are known to suppress immunity
- infection(s) with CMV (cytomegalovirus)
- infection(s) with "other sexually transmitted pathogens."

When these elements are combined, both cellular and humoral factors join to impair the CMV-killing ability of cytotoxic white cells. The invading virus then gains the upper hand and proliferates, bringing about further suppression of immunity due to biomechanical changes having "positive feedback systems" (Sonnabend and Saadoun 1984).

SYMPTOMS

The expression of AIDS follows two characteristic patterns: the presence of unusual *opportunistic infections* that normally do not get through a competent immune system; and the presence of otherwise *rare cancers* (such as KS).

Minor symptoms may precede these severe symptoms, including several that are also symptoms of many other afflictions. These minor symptoms include: swollen lymph glands, a weight loss of 10 percent or more of body weight (discounting dieting and exercise loss), fatigue and malaise for more than a week, fever and sweats, abnormal bleeding, skin rash (or rash inside the mouth, nose, or anus), persistent diarrhea, shortness of breath and/or coughing, and headache and confusion. Onset of these symptoms usually precedes the diagnosis of AIDS by three to six months.

AIDS is a complex of many diseases. Some of the characteristic diseases and infectious organisms are listed in Table 14.

AIDS AND THE IMMUNE RESPONSE

Most AIDS victims have a history of multiple insults to their immune systems. J. M. Reuben and coworkers (1983) performed an immunological characterization of homosexual males. They found that all of their subjects had a history of multiple sex part-

TABLE 14

Characteristic Diseases and Infections Associated with AIDS

Organism or Disease	Infection Site	Symptoms
Bacteria		
Mycobacterium avium intra-cellularae	Liver, lymph nodes, spleen, bone marrow, lung	Fever, malaise, swollen glands, sweats, liver function abnormalities, cough, sputum
Pulmonary nocardiosis	Lung	Fever, cough, shortness of breath, bloody sputum, pain in breathing
Salmonella	Intestine, blood stream	Diarrhea, cramps, fever, sweats, skin rash, chills
Shigella flexneri	Intestine	Diarrhea, cramps, bloody stools, fever
Legionella pneumophilia	Lung	Fever, cough, shortness of breath
Fungi		
Candida albicans		
1. Mucocutaneous	Mouth, esophagus	White spots in mouth, especially tongue; tenderness and pain in gums and teeth; difficulty swallowing
2. Disseminated	Blood, liver, kidneys, brain	Fever, chills, sweats, confusion, somnolence, wasting, liver function abnormalities
Cryptococcus neoformans	Skin, brain, lung	Headache, dizziness, stiff neck, confusion, coma, shortness of breath, cough, fever
Aspergillosis	Lung, brain	Fever, cough, bloody sputum, confusion, headache, seizures
Histoplasmosis	Lung, lymph nodes, skin	Fever, cough, sweats, weight loss, swollen glands, rash
Protozoa		
Pneumocystis carinii	Lung	Fever, cough, shortness of breath; white, foamy sputum
Toxoplasma gondii	Brain, central nervous system, lymph nodes, blood	Confusion, headache, seizures, dizziness, swollen glands, fever, malaise
Cryptosporidium enteritis	Intestine	Severe, watery diarrhea
Isospora belli	Intestine	Severe, watery diarrhea
Giardia lamblia	Intestine	Diarrhea, food intolerance, flatulence, nausea, cramps

Organism or Disease	Infection Site	Symptoms
Entamoeba histolytica	Intestine, liver	Diarrhea, food intolerance, flatulence, nausea, cramps, bloody stool, jaundice, liver function abnormalities
Viruses (or suspected viral diseases)		
Cytomegalovirus (CMV)	Lung, lymph nodes, liver, blood	Cough, shortness of breath, fever, swollen glands, jaundice, abdominal pain
Epstein-Barr	Lymph nodes, liver, blood, central nervous system	Fever, swollen glands, jaundice, liver function abnormalities, abdominal pain, confusion, nerve palsy
Herpes simplex	Skin of mouth, hands, genitals, buttocks, brain	Confusion, coma, fever, seizures, skin sores, swollen glands
Hepatitis B	Liver, joints	Jaundice, fever, food and alcohol intolerance, dark urine, light stool, joint pain and swelling
Multifocal leukoencephalopathy	Brain	Confusion, seizures, lethargy, coma
Subacute sclerosing panencephalitis	Brain	Confusion, seizures, lethargy, coma

Source: Mayer and Pizer, 1983

ners, multiple sexually transmitted diseases, and mild to moderate viral, bacterial, parasitic, or fungal infections. All had used "recreational" drugs. Healthy active homosexual males have reduced T helper to suppressor ratios compared to healthy active heterosexuals (Detels et al. 1983; Reuben et al. 1983; Kornfeld et al. 1982). This lowered helper to suppressor ratio is due to elevated levels of suppressor cells. Individuals with AIDS have a lowered helper to suppressor ratio. (Refer back to Chapter 2 for a discussion of helper to suppressor ratios.)

Sexually active homosexual men, hemophiliacs, and intravenous drug users all have a high incidence of having had hepatitis B infection at some time in their lives. Hepatitis B is a known immunosuppressant and is thought to be transmitted through bodily fluids.

A new form of hepatitis has been documented that has the potential of becoming more deadly than existing forms. Known as delta hepatitis, the disease agent responsible consists of a new virus on the inside combined with the surface antigen portion of the hepatitis B virus around it. This disease can infect only people who already have hepatitis B. Both infections can occur simultaneously, which makes the potential for fatality much greater. Delta infection can also change a mild form of hepatitis B infection into a very damaging illness, even cirrhosis.

Blood and blood-product transfusion, especially those from blood derivatives obtained from thousands of donors, are key risk factors. In Mediterranean countries, delta infection is found among people with hepatitis B and is probably transmitted by intimate contact (N. S. Nishioka and J. L. Dienstag, 1985, *New England Journal of Medicine* 312(23): 1515).

SPERM AND IMMUNOSUPPRESSION

Another piece of the disease puzzle is that human seminal plasma produces immune suppression (James and Cullen 1983). Some researchers believe that spermatozoa themselves can suppress immunity.

The biological "reason" for this activity is to enable sperm to travel through "hostile" territory, the female reproductive tract. Here, sperm are "seen" as antigens and must fight against antibodies produced in the female, to protect against these foreign invaders.

When a man repeatedly exposes himself to *different* sperm (that is, many sexual partners), it is as though he is confronting many different antigens. This is thought to be a predisposing factor for AIDS, owing to the formation of "antibodies which cross react with lymphoid cells" and *circulating immune complexes,* or CICs. Homosexuals who contract AIDS frequently show both of these components (sperm antibodies and CICs) in their blood. Unfortunately, homosexuals *not* manifesting this disease all too frequently also show these telltale signs of latent infection (Witkin, Bongiovanni, and Yu 1983).

Experiments where healthy male rabbits were rectally inseminated weekly with semen pooled from other rabbits showed the presence of CICs, sperm antibodies, and other markers of this specific immune reaction.

Spermatozoa, then, provoke immune responses, and in a susceptible person can bring on the full-blown disease syndrome. By altering mechanisms of immune regulation, circulating CICs and antibodies thus markedly increase the likelihood of infection. Simply put, there is much evidence that sperm itself suppresses immunity (Rodman, Laurence, and Pruslin 1985). When it is injected into the anus, which is not adapted to receive such an assault of antigenlike bodies, coupled with the suspected AIDS virus, the disease process may be initiated.

PREVENTION

The common sense ways to avoid or control AIDS are discussed below. In addition to their anti-AIDS value, these measures are prudent for preventing a variety of illnesses — in particular, the sexually transmitted diseases.

Bolster your immunocompetence with protective foods and specific vitamin and mineral supplements (see Chapters 5 and 6), rest, exercise, and mental conditioning (see Chapters 4 and 7). It is reasonable to believe that if your immune system is properly stimulated, you may come in contact with the suspected AIDS virus without contracting the disease. Stimulating immunity is your primary *defensive* measure regarding AIDS. The remainder of the suggestions here consist of *avoidance* techniques to reduce your chances of *exposure* to AIDS.

Limit the number of people with whom you have sexual contact, especially encounters of the "one-night-stand" variety. This not only protects you from elevated contact risk, it also enables you to contact your partner(s) should you develop the disease.

Do not use intravenous drugs and avoid sexual contact with intravenous drug users. This does not mean that diabetics should not inject themselves with insulin (which is via the subcutaneous route). The danger is not present in a sterile needle; it comes from sharing a needle with another, infected individual or from using a contaminated needle.

To control disease spread, if you *do* use intravenous drugs, have multiple sex partners, or suspect that you may have come in contact with AIDS, *do not donate blood*. It has been shown that infants, hemophiliacs, and other blood transfusion recipients have acquired AIDS through donated blood products from infected individuals.

If a sexual partner appears to be ill, avoid sexual contact until the illness has been diagnosed. However, the incubation period of AIDS may be up to five years, and sexual contact with a suspected AIDS carrier — no matter how healthy the person may look — should be approached with caution.

Observe good hygiene practices such as washing any portion of your body that may have come in contact with either a fluid or mucous membrane of a suspected AIDS carrier. Also, do not rub your eyes after handling fluids of an AIDS patient. The pathogen may enter your body through any available opening. (The suspected virus is extremely sensitive to soap and water, chlorine, even heat, and is easily destroyed.)

Avoid anal intercourse. Passive (receptive) individuals seem to have lower T helper to suppressor ratio levels than the active (insertive) individuals (Detels et al. 1983). The reason for this difference is unknown. One hypothesis is that in the passive partner the rectal mucosa becomes torn, allowing the entrance of semen, bacteria, feces, etc., into the body. Similarly, other activities involving oral-anal and manual-anal contact will result in a similar increased risk factor.

Sexually active people should undergo regular medical checkups to detect and treat sexually transmitted diseases before they do too much damage to the body and the immune system.

Do not use "recreational" drugs such as "poppers" (nitrite inhalant drugs used frequently in the gay community to heighten sexual pleasure). Poppers have been shown to be immunosuppressive agents in mice. If they have the same effect in humans, their use could leave you more susceptible to attack by opportunistic pathogens.

THIS DISEASE MAY NOT BE FATAL!

One very promising regimen for treating AIDS is being administered by Robert F. Cathcart III, M.D., in Los Altos, California. Dr. Cathcart has treated more people for serious viral illnesses (hepatitis, mononucleosis, viral pneumonia, even the common cold) employing vitamin C than anyone else — more than twelve thousand patients!

As he had expected, Dr. Cathcart has found that vitamin C, in the form of ascorbate, is very valuable for treating AIDS patients when used in conjunction with certain conventional treatments.

News of the ascorbate treatment is spreading rapidly among communities at high risk for AIDS. Ascorbate is being used by an increasing percentage of the AIDS patient population, but without much guidance and often without the knowledge of their physicians. For this reason, Dr. Cathcart has written a preliminary protocol to help physicians treat their AIDS patients with this helpful vitamin.

His preliminary recommendations are based upon the anecdotal reports of some ninety AIDS patients who were treated by physicians but who also took high doses of ascorbate on their own, as well as twelve AIDS patients treated by Dr. Cathcart himself.

The following article is our condensation of Dr. Cathcart's protocol for treating AIDS and AIDS-related conditions.

VITAMIN C TREATMENT PROTOCOL FOR AIDS

By Robert F. Cathcart III, M.D.

As predicted, AIDS patients are usually capable of ingesting large doses of ascorbate. It is desirable that the amount of ascorbate taken orally be maximized. Patients are *titrated to bowel tolerance* (the amount that almost but not quite causes diarrhea). A *balanced ascorbate* mixture is utilized which is made up of a mixture of approximately 25 percent buffered ascorbate salts (calcium, magnesium, and potassium ascorbate) and 75 percent ascorbic acid. This mixture is dissolved in a small amount of water and taken at least every hour. The purpose of the frequent doses and this balanced mixture is to maximize the amount of ascorbate tolerated without producing diarrhea. The usual amount tolerated initially is between 40 and 100 grams per 24 hours. Doses in excess of 100 grams per 24 hours may be necessary temporarily with secondary bacterial and viral infections. As the patient's condition improves, bowel tolerance will decrease.

If oral solutions of ascorbate are used over a long period of time, care should be taken to keep them off the teeth by using a straw in order to avoid enamel damage.

When intravenous ascorbate is found necessary because the patient is unable to take adequate amounts of ascorbate to scavenge all of the free radicals created by AIDS and the various secondary infections, the following intravenous treatments should be utilized. Sodium ascorbate buffered to a pH of 7.4 and without preservatives is added to sterile water in a concentration of 60 grams per 500 cc. (For patients with small veins, the concentration should be 60 grams per liter.)

The infusions should be given over at least a three-hour period, preferably longer. Daily administration of three bottles, 180 grams per 24 hours, may be necessary in acutely ill patients. Enough should be administered to detoxify the patient regardless of the amount. Additionally, oral doses of ascorbate should be taken simultaneously with the intravenous ascorbate.

It is absolutely essential that the patient's intestinal parasites are treated in the conventional manner. *Entamoeba histolytica*, especially, and *Giardia lamblia* must be treated, as well as other intestinal parasites not ordinarily considered pathogenic. Herxheimer's reactions [a temporary worsening of symptoms, owing to the release of toxins from dying parasites] should be expected frequently. Symptoms including Kaposi's may be exacerbated, despite the ascorbate, during treatment for intestinal parasites.

Candida also should be sought and treated. Patients owe it to themselves and society to treat the Candida consistently, because of the possibility of breeding resistant strains. In patients who clinically appear to have Candida but in whom Candida cannot be cultured, sensitivities to Candida should be suspected and treatment of especially the bowel should be considered. In these sensitive patients, foods and vitamins containing yeasts should be avoided. Lactobacillus in large amounts should be fed to these patients. [See Chapter 13 for more information on candidiasis.]

Bacterial infections should be treated with appropriate antibiotics but large amounts of Lactobacillus should be administered with foods if there is the slightest tendency to Candida infections or sensitivities. Ascorbate administration should be intensified during treatment for bacterial infections. Intravenous ascorbate may be necessary.

Viral infections should be treated with intensification of the ascorbate treatment. Intravenous ascorbate may become necessary. Herpes infections may benefit from a paste of ascorbate and water applied four times a day directly to the lesions starting when the patient first perceives an impending attack.

Immunosuppressive therapy should *not* be utilized.

Sugar and processed foods, foods with chemicals, recreational drugs, cigarettes, alcohol, etc. should be avoided. Obvious nutritional deficits should be sought and corrected.

Food sensitivities are common because of the disorders of the immune system, and often account for apparent adverse reactions to vitamin C. Skin rashes and gastrointestinal discomforts may occur, but are almost never due to the ascorbate itself. Most ascorbate is made from corn. Residuals of corn or chemicals used in manufacturing the ascorbate are almost invariably the cause of the sensitivity reactions. Ascorbates made from sago palm or from tapioca are often tolerated. Different brands should be tried. It is almost always possible to find some ascorbate that is tolerated. This sensitivity problem is very important to deal with because patients frequently feel their life depends on taking adequate amounts of ascorbate, and they may be correct in this feeling.

All sharing of body fluids and fecal material should stop. Repeated exposures, not only to possible AIDS infection, but to the secondary infections, especially intestinal parasites and Candida should be avoided.

With this protocol, it may be anticipated that a large percentage of patients will slowly go into an extended clinical remission. Patients must be on guard to sense any impending infection, colds, etc. The patient should begin the additional large frequent doses of ascorbate within minutes of such diagnosis.

Dr. Cathcart's work is of paramount importance, yet the research establishment refuses to fund his nutritional-biochemical AIDS treatment research plan. Interested readers may write to Dr. Cathcart c/o Fund for Ethnic Medicine, Box 183, Fairfax, CA 94930, and receive his complete protocol for treating AIDS.

EIGHTEEN CASES IN REMISSION!

While their stories do not generally make the news, other health professionals have also been able to achieve significant remissions in AIDS cases, using nontraditional approaches. The program described below uses bowel-tolerance doses of vitamin C, based on Dr. Cathcart's regimen, while also incorporating other modalities of healing. The physician Russ Jaffe, M.D., Ph.D., is also a brilliant biochemist with experience as a researcher at the National Institutes of Health. Despite this impressive background and hard data regarding *surviving patients,* the medical establishment ignores his nutritional, psychological, and physical therapeutic program. Instead, nearly fifty million dollars will be spent this year on looking for an elusive virus, defining new diagnostic methodology, locating new "cases" worldwide, and exploring the same dead-end drugs used for years in cancer treatment.

I interviewed Dr. Jaffe in Mill Valley, California, some time before he presented his paper at the annual meeting of the Orthomolecular Medical Society in February 1985 in San Francisco. Through the protocol described in this interview, a group of health professionals has achieved remission in a small group of eighteen AIDS patients for more than eighteen months.

INTERVIEW WITH RUSS JAFFE, M.D., PH.D.

MW: How do you know that these patients had AIDS, and how do you know that they "remissed" from AIDS?

RJ: The diagnosis of AIDS was based on the CDC [Centers for Disease Control] definition. [This definition includes details concerning laboratory values for various immune functions.] As part of that definition, new infections are often met with a significantly *weak* antibody response, even though the B cells appear otherwise normal. Thus infection with intestinal or systemic protozoa such as *Pneumocystis carinii,* with fungi such as candida, with viruses or bacteria, are not surprising. These infectious agents are generally of low infectivity and virulence, but in the susceptible host they can be life threatening.

The basic message is that the hazard of AIDS derives from a possibly avoidable set of consequences, rather than from the primary condition itself. And, while a viral etiology is under active investigation, the *predisposition* or susceptibility to that virus may also be important.

In addition, a *nonmalignant tumor,* named for the pathologist who first described it, Dr. Kaposi, is often present. A malignant condition, lymphoma, is sometimes present.

The majority of our patients — fourteen out of eighteen — presented initially with Kaposi's tumor. However, their immune functions become progressively depressed as they are followed, and these Kaposi's patients often subsequently develop opportunistic infections. Also, patients who presented initially with infections may later develop Kaposi's tumors.

Pneumocystis carinii infection or Kaposi's sarcoma, or both, without other obvious cause for adult acquired immunosuppression, is highly suggestive of AIDS. In addition we had T and B cell, helper, suppressor, killer, and null cell analyses done by various laboratories. These patients all had a ratio of helper to suppressor cells of less than 0.2, and most showed ratios of 0.1.

This is *half* the level of the ratio that is considered by CDC to be characteristic of adult acquired immunodeficiency.

So these were nineteen really immunodeficient men, eleven of whom developed *Pneumocystis carinii* and fourteen of whom had Kaposi's sarcoma. Now, it is important to be aware that at the National Institutes of Health, Jose Costa has shown that *Kaposi's sarcoma is not cancer.** It is a benign tumor, an overgrowth of normal epithelial cells around very delicate, electrically active nerve bundles.

It is not a sarcoma, not a cancer, and it *should not be treated with chemotherapy!* Spontaneous remission makes sense if you establish regulatory control. The body would melt away the cells; they're rapidly dividing epithelial cells — they rapidly divide and rapidly die. And if they stop growing they won't divide.

MW: So the patients you worked with were principally patients with KS?

RJ: No. Fourteen KS and eleven *Pneumocystis carinii.* All nineteen to get into the study had to have a less than 0.2 ratio of helper to suppressor cells. In fact, the median was 0.1. This is sickness near unto death! Now, a year later roughly, the median is around 0.4 — from 0.1 to 0.4.

MW: That's still not too high.

RJ: You want it to be 2? [Two, or 0.8, is the average normal helper to suppressor ratio.] In only one year, what do you want from me? From 0.1 to 0.4 is a big improvement. Some of them are up to 2.

MW: Who diagnoses remission?

RJ: The same doctor that diagnoses the disease, and not a member of our study team. This is not a "self-fulfilling prophecy."

The diagnosis of remission is based on the change in lymphocyte ratio. It's up fourfold, from 0.1 to 0.4. And it's over 0.2 [the CDC "cut-off" separating the significantly at risk from the moderately at risk].

MW: How do you look at the development of AIDS, from a clinical standpoint?

RJ: Basically, you dig yourself into a hole by a combination of lifestyle choices, and some people are able, fortunately, to dig themselves out of it. I'm telling them, "It's going to take you two to three years to recover," and some people are willing to follow a program of health enhancement based on our suggestions.

MW: Now, they have to be sustained, don't they, Russ?

RJ: Of course. Frankly, we believe and we tell the patients that they should be meticulous and follow each aspect of the program. Compliance is important, as with any medical, therapeutic intervention. We recommend that support groups be started by small clusters of patients — say, ten to fifteen. These groups are self-organized, self-paced, and self-sustained. This is entirely an option taken by patients, with our encouragement. They allow them to talk with each other and have a sense of community, a sense of belonging. Some have volunteered to peer counselors that the group is the most significant relationship in their life. Some have reported a spontaneous change in "compulsive sexuality," and some have found "peer co-counseling" of significant benefit.

MW: Now, let's go back to the question of compliance on the part of the patient.

RJ: It is our impression that it is very important. For example, a rule of thumb which I tell patients is that they should be extremely honest in their communication. "No time for B.S." is the way some of us put it.

   What we have to offer clinically is limited. However, we can offer them hope. We can offer them *hopefulness*. We can offer them *helpfulness*.

MW: Who is this "us" you keep referring to?

RJ: At one level, it is an "invisible university" or network of clinical researchers, policy planners, futurists, strategic planners, theorists, practitioners, etc. At another level it is an entrepreneurial activity by a biomedical laboratory.

MW: How do you help people to increase their awareness of the reality of their situation and constructive options with which to deal with it?

RJ: What we do is recommend a menu of self-awareness improvement techniques that are self-paced and self-actualizing. For example, we encourage active meditation.

MW: What can you tell the readers about the program you recommend?

RJ: It is typically a seven- or eight-faceted program. The first thing is: identify and case in a positive light the "image of reality" or the "image of the self" that the person has of themselves.

MW: So it's psychotherapeutic, then?

RJ: No! It is *therapeutic*. By this we mean, we do not find the Cartesian division of *mind* and *body* to be more than useful organizing principles in the study of human development. From a clinical point of view, anything that affects your mind influences your body and anything that affects your body has a reciprocal effect on your perception of mind.

We are *mind;* we are *body;* and, perhaps, we are even more than that. In any event, we are clearly interconnected.

MW: Now . . . back to the specific suggestions you make.

RJ: Broadly, they can be summarized as:

1. Learn new patterns of consumption; this must be individualized

2. Take balanced, nonirritating supplements

3. Drink adequate amounts of "good for you" fluid

4. Exercise appropriately for you

5. Cultivate a relaxation reflex to reduce the cost of "stress"

6. Breathe efficiently

7. Commit to expressing health in your life.

MW: Can you rephrase this for our readers?

RJ: With pleasure:

1. You are OK. You can express this by the foods you eat; the liquids you drink; the way you consume and process stress; the way you consume and process relationships; the way you consume attitudes about yourself.

2. Take vitamins, minerals, essential fats, lecithins, amino acids, adaptogens, or whatever it is that your body needs more of than it is getting. Of course, this must be carefully monitored. More is not necessarily better. Optimums may vary widely from person to person and from time to time.

3. Drink uncontaminated water; drink fruit juice; drink vegetable juice; drink fresh vegetable broth; drink consommé; drink bouillon; drink herbal beverages; drink citrus juices; drink soup, etc.

4. Exercise your body; "work your body"; improve the mechanical efficiency of your human machine. This might involve swimming, hiking, running, climbing, aerobics, trampolining, etc.

5. Allow a relaxation response — what some people call a "relaxation reflex," a quieting reflex — to become part of your every-

day existence. For example, read *Active Meditation* by Drs. Robert Leichtman and Carl Japikse.

6. Learn to breathe more effectively. For example, read *The Science of Breath* by Dr. Rudolph Ballantine.

7. If you visualize yourself as healthy and do this from a significant internal need and with a quiet confidence that what you want is for the good of the situation, if you are willing to be honest with yourself and with those around you, at least we know that it will not do you any harm. And, it may help significantly. Here, again, the book by Dr. Leichtman [cited above] is helpful. The work of Dr. Carl Simonton and his wife, Stephanie, [*Getting Well Again*], along with that of Dr. Jerry Jampolsky [*Love Is Letting Go of Fear*], is noteworthy.

And there are always personal details. Items that are distinctive to the needs, desires, and perceptions of the patient are always important. So is the "chemistry" of the professional and the client. We in the profession call it "bedside or deskside manner."

MW: What about the psychosocial aspects of patients with AIDS?

RJ: Here I am not really equipped to answer. My background is in clinical and basic research. This does not professionally equip me to answer questions about psychosocial aspects of a given condition. I will, however, offer a personal opinion. Part of the reason the support groups may be so important is that, once diagnosed, people are often subjected to humiliating loss of friends, loved ones, work, social contacts, and the like. This happens often. There has been, and sometimes, there continues to be, hysterical misunderstanding about the risk of contacting a patient with AIDS. This is the same thing that used to be in regard to TB, leprosy, hepatitis, and cancer. Fortunately, most of us are more mature and compassionate.

As a general rule, healthy people are not susceptible to infectious agents — and this includes the HTLV-III or similar virus.

MW: Do you think that AIDS is communicable?

RJ: No . . . and maybe. No; I do not believe that healthy people will get AIDS. On the other hand, compromised hosts are at greater risk of acquiring infections and this includes AIDS. So, my suggestion is that we all keep our health quotient up and our disease quotient down; enjoy more and worry less; be prudent but enjoy life.

MW: Easy for you to say that.

RJ: And easy to live that way, once you make the commitment.
Those of us who take health seriously and take the enjoyment of
life seriously find that we have more time and energy to pursue
our interests because of the time and effort devoted to the maintenance of excellent health.

Health is easier to maintain than it is to acquire — just like
the other significant possessions in our lives. If we make the investment in health, tangible reward is probable. The amount of
investment required depends on your constitution and your lifestyle.*

Dr. Jaffe's experience with his AIDS patients is a powerful confirmation of the principles of immune protection we spelled out in
Chapters 4 through 7 of this book.

IS AIDS COMMUNICABLE?

There is no question that AIDS is an epidemic that is consistently
on the upward spiral. The number of reported cases is increasing
rapidly among known risk groups, yet political considerations
block the drastic public health measures that are necessary to
confront the disease.

When cholera was found to be transmitted by contaminated
water supplies, public wells were closed. Swamps are drained to
eliminate mosquito breeding grounds in malaria zones. Why are
gay bath houses still open for business as usual? Why do newspa-
pers continue to carry advertisements that extol orgiastic behavior?

As for the direct communicability of AIDS, we must say that
the opinion of experts we have interviewed is definitely "no." It is
not likely that *casual* contact with a person actively harboring the
suspected virus will result in transmission of the disease. You
should remember, however, that a susceptible or immune-compromised person has an increased chance of contracting *any* disease. It is also worth noting that viruses have been kept alive
outside the human body for up to eight hours. Colds, influenza,

---

*Dr. Jaffe's view, while not shared by all physicians, is generally accepted by
members of the Orthomolecular Medical Society, a group of innovative clinicians.

hepatitis, mononucleosis, even AIDS viruses are theoretically transmissible via public telephones, public restrooms, restaurants, or other "disease merry-go-rounds." A person with a suppressed immune system *could* pick up any of the causative viruses through these passive routes, which is why immune enhancement is emphasized in this book and especially in this chapter.

On heterosexual AIDS. The evidence, to date, does *not* show a rapid spread of this disease into the heterosexual population. According to one expert, Dr. John Seale, a genitourinary specialist, formerly with the Middlesex and St. Thomas Hospital in London, "the organism (virus) is not known to penetrate the cell walls of undamaged genital cells, or to replicate within those cells and be released into the blood, or to shed large quantities of infectious particles into genital secretions." As reported in the February 14, 1985, issue of *New Scientist,* Dr. Seale goes on to suggest that anal intercourse is a key requirement for sexual transmission. This is due to the fact that the rectal wall is only one cell thick, and the skin of the penis is so vulnerable that even slight abrasions would permit viral transmission from one sexual partner to another. Those homosexuals who engage in frequent sex with many different partners, or those who engage in a practice known as "fisting" (inserting the hand through the anus into the large bowel and then forming a fist), are at the highest risk for this disease. It makes sense that such practices would increase the risk of spreading the suspected virus, because such behavior opens the rectum to viral transmission and, from there, brings the virus directly into the blood stream. The bowel is clearly not adapted to receive any kind of foreign material through the anus, but to excrete, or get rid of waste products. By going against nature in such a profound manner, only harm can follow.

But what about women who engage in anal-genital sexual practices with men? Do they contract AIDS? So far we do not know. Of the relatively few women who have contracted this disease, almost all have reported they lived with men who were intravenous drug users. They were not asked about the specifics of their sex with men. (Obviously my statement does not refer to the tragic deaths of several women who contracted the disease through blood transfusions. The eighty-year-old grandmother and the suburban housewife who died in the San Francisco area

unfortunately received tainted blood transfusions.) Following this
question of AIDS among women, scientists are looking at sexual
practices among African women, because there, many women appear with the disease. Should anal-genital sex, or bisexual practices prove to be more common in Africa, it would tend to support
the theory that anal sex is a key factor in this disease.

Also of importance are the issues of scarification, mentioned
earlier as a common practice in Haiti, and tattooing. Both practices open the skin to infection and pass blood from one person to
another if the needles used are not sterilized between use. (My
thanks to James Scanlon, a writer for the *Coastal Post,* Bolinas,
California, for sharing with me his article on heterosexual AIDS.)

For the present, the best advice for any sexually active person is
to strictly limit the number of sexual partners (preferably to one),
not to engage in anal sex, and to use common sanitation such as
soap and water before and after engaging. This is not "moralistic"
preaching, but advice based on current knowledge of this night-
marish epidemic.

What about secondary infectiousness? On a recent radio talk
show, a woman who called in said, "My brother is gay and has
AIDS. I'm pregnant and I'm going to deliver in a few weeks. Is it
safe for my brother to visit?" The host answered, "Absolutely,
yes."

Well, that may be true, as far as AIDS is concerned — that the
brother is not likely to spread AIDS. But the problem is that
AIDS patients have lost their cellular immunity, which would do
such things as kill fungus; kill parasites; kill bacteria; kill intracellular viruses, as opposed to extracellular ones; and kill off cancer
cells. That is why AIDS patients have repeated problems with infections. You do not find the AIDS patient simply catching cold
more than anyone else — that is primarily an extracellular type of
viral infection. What the AIDS patient gets is herpes, chronic
hepatitis, and other serious infectious diseases.

So, the pregnant woman and the embryo may not be at risk for
AIDS, but very well might be for the other organisms and diseases
that this particular AIDS patient possibly harbors.

AIDS is a major public health problem, and political decisions
will not change the behavior of a virus, fungus, bacterium, or
protozoan. Stronger controls, both within and outside high-risk

groups, are needed. Even though there is now encouraging evidence that AIDS *is* curable, as we have seen in this chapter, *prevention* — both personal and public — is the wisest and least costly course.

CONTROLLING AIDS

In addition to following the recommendations already given, we have to face the difficult problems that demand resolution. I realize the sensitive nature of some of the proposals I am about to make, but these may be the wisest courses of action open to us. By arguing the question, or trying to hide from the facts, we only *increase* the gravity of the problem and risk greatly increasing the number of patients, which may lead to measures that will border on the outright fascistic.

First, it is advisable to establish *separate hospitals,* one in the New York City area and one in the San Francisco area, for the treatment of diagnosed AIDS patients. This will contain the spread from accidental causes that are hospital related, give patients the best care possible, and allow volunteers to work in a selected environment. Having a physician traveling from an AIDS ward to an obstetrics ward, as is now the case in some hospitals, is equivalent to the days when doctors performed autopsies and then rushed to deliver a child without scrubbing! It is only a matter of time before hospital-transmitted diseases will begin to appear in "nonrisk" patients, so separate hospitals are a rational course to follow.

As pointed out earlier, while AIDS may not be casually transmitted, the *secondary infections* are transmissable, especially in a hospital where people already have lowered immunity to disease. AIDS patients have lost their cellular immunity and, therefore, may be harboring the organisms for viral, bacterial, fungal, and parasitic infections. We want to reduce the risk of spreading these infections, and separate hospitals for AIDS patients is one means for doing this.

Second, developing a simple test for the presence of the AIDS *antigen* (that is, the causative virus) must be given the highest priority. The present test for *antibodies* to the suspected AIDS virus is not very useful as a preventive tool. It may show "positive" for an individual who has already mounted an attack against the virus, survived, and is at little risk of coming down with AIDS.* It may show "negative" for a person who has just come in contact with the virus and has not yet developed antibodies, yet who *will* contract the disease in the future. The test for the AIDS antigen, once developed, should be administered as part of a *national mandatory screening program.*

By conducting such a test on a national scale, we can then devote our public health efforts to educating those "positives" about how to *raise their resistance* using techniques outlined in this book. By reporting periodically for T cell counts, and other markers of immune system function, those at risk will know where they stand at each step of the process and be able to decide what they want to do about their state of health. This sequence will protect both "at-risk" individuals (those positive for the AIDS antigen) and the general population.

The issue of civil liberties must be faced, so the politics of AIDS is not allowed to continue to dominate public health decisions for containing this disease.

In an epidemic as virulent as this one is, emergency measures are called for. To protect the population, we must all agree to cooperate. The screening I suggest is *not* limited to any single group or groups. It is recommended that the entire national population be tested.

The third measure for containing this epidemic is to cease disseminating the idea that there is such a thing as "safe sex" for the group at greatest risk, male homosexuals. "Deep" kissing a carrier of the suspected AIDS virus can spread the infectious organism when it is present, and we have no definitive way of knowing if it is present until the person develops a case of the disease!

Fourth, we must make it clear that we want at least 50 percent of all AIDS-associated money† spent on evaluating the reported success of *nonconventional therapies* in bringing about remissions in

---

*A recent study found that many people in eastern Zaire who are positive for the HTLV-III antibody show *no* signs of immunosuppression and are perfectly healthy.

†In 1985 almost ninety-three million dollars were spent on AIDS in the U.S. alone. Of this only 4 percent was spent on "public information," and even this information did little more than tell people to practice "safe sex." Stronger constraints are necessary to control this epidemic.

AIDS patients. At this time, the best the conventional medical world has to offer is both very expensive and 100 percent fatal!

THE POLITICS OF AIDS

It is interesting that both spectrums of the political world have refused to publish an independent view of the AIDS epidemic. *The National Review,* a "conservative" periodical, and *The New Republic,* a "liberal" periodical, both rejected my offer to present the latest data regarding this disease. I suspect that the "right" does not want to acknowledge that there *is* a major problem while their favorite son is in office, while the "left" would have us believe this disease is quite democratic and strikes all groups equally, without regard to lifestyle.

The reason we are hearing about the dangers of AIDS spreading into the "general" population can be traced to propagandists in the homosexual community and certain researchers who stand to gain more funding if the disease is seen as a general threat. (Apparently, this alarmist note was rung by some members of the AIDS Medical Foundation, according to a recent article in a homosexual-oriented newspaper. This stratagem backfired, of course, even causing one of the cofounders to resign in protest from the scientific committee. See *New York Native,* October 7–13, 1985, p. 25.) But generalizing the risk and setting off an alarm reaction in the general population has had an effect opposite to the one desired by those who wish to generate sympathy for people with AIDS. People now tend to blame the *known* risk groups for spreading this infection. This will *increase* the pariahlike status of homosexuals, bisexuals, and intravenous drug users, not the amount of sympathy. Second, research funding is likely to be *decreased* by groups calling for spending the money to quarantine patients and those in known risk groups. Third, vigilante action is likely to be unleashed should unthinking mobs be led to believe they are at risk for this disease.

For these reasons, I hope the facts about AIDS are made known as widely as possible, both in the United States and throughout other countries where the disease is spreading. By altering risky behavior and learning which nutrients are immune enhancing, all of us can stimulate our natural resistance to this and other diseases, while those at risk for AIDS or those diagnosed with the disease can avail themselves of the alternative therapies that show great promise.

Homosexual activists have claimed that much "disinformation" about how AIDS is spread is being promulgated to "punish" their cohorts. It would be wiser for them to accept the blame for bringing this disease to present levels and to acknowledge that AIDS is primarily a disease of male homosexuals. By putting one's own house in order, the world sometimes follows suit. It is true that attitudes and behavior are rapidly changing among responsible homosexual men, but these people were never in the group at highest risk. Those who practice orgiastic sex, with many partners, and use street drugs are not likely to respond to reason. (One clinician, who asked to remain anonymous, told us that several AIDS patients returned to "bath houses" for anonymous sex each time their symptoms diminished!)

Freedom is not license, which our human rights activists have failed to realize. The rights of the overall population are also to be protected. By protecting only the sick or the handicapped — that is, by attempting to bring the entire society to a single common denominator — we may eliminate the healthiest from protection. Magistrates in England have faced this problem and have decided they have the right to hospitalize people diagnosed with AIDS, whether or not the patient so desires. By allowing such very sick people to come and go as they please as outpatients, we may actually be encouraging the spread of this disease.

Having said what has not been said publicly (by health officials, who voice similar concerns privately), I must reiterate my appeal for compassion and first-rate treatment for the sufferers of this horrible complex of diseases. The purpose in trying to isolate causes, be they lifestyle associated, political, or sociological, is not to lay blame but to move rapidly to stem the spread and treat the patients. All of us will agree that these are the goals of any rational public health program.

∘ 11 ∘

Self Against Self: The Autoimmune Diseases

AN ELDERLY WOMAN, walking bent over, holding a cane, every step painful because of her rheumatoid arthritis; a young child giving himself an insulin injection for his diabetes; a roomful of adults, mostly women, giving each other support in coping with their shared disease, lupus — these people may appear to have little in common, but in fact all are suffering from a group of diverse and often mysterious disorders that have all been labeled "autoimmune diseases." A properly functioning immune system protects the body against invading antigens, but in the case of the autoimmune diseases, the body turns against itself, with the immune defenses attacking the cells and tissues of the body they are supposed to protect.

In an autoimmune disease, the body begins producing *autoantigens* (its own antigens!), to which it responds by producing autoantibodies. Any part of the immune system may go haywire in this way. The problem may be with the T cells, or with antibody production, or with both.

Usually the immune system ignores normal body components with which it is familiar. Why, then, would it begin perceiving such components as enemies? There are several theories to account for this. The autoantigen may be a normal body component, but one that is not usually present in the circulation; and so, it may not be recognized when it does appear. Autoantibodies may arise from chemical, physical, or biological alterations of normal body cells. Or, body cells may bear some resemblance to foreign antigens, and so be attacked along with the foreign cells. Another possibility is that the fighting cells of the immune system may undergo a mutation, causing them to attack normal body components.

All these theories are based on the supposition that autoimmune diseases are due to *overactivity* on the part of the immune system. However, this may be an oversimplification, since autoimmune diseases are actually much more common among people with immune deficiencies — that is, people whose immune systems are *under*active. For example, rheumatoid arthritis, an autoimmune disease, is thirty times more common among people with Bruton's syndrome, an immune deficiency disease, than it is among the general population.

The role of genetic factors in autoimmune diseases is unknown at present. Besides genetics, there may also be a strong environmental component that serves as the trigger. One possible trigger is pathogenic organisms. In one study, laboratory animals whose immune systems had been suppressed at a very early age, if raised in a germ-free environment were not found to develop autoimmune diseases until late in life, if at all. Others, raised in a normal, nonsterile environment, developed symptoms identical to human autoimmune disease conditions (Fudenberg 1971). Other environmental factors, besides micro-organisms, that may trigger autoimmune diseases are drugs (including penicillin, antihypertensive and anticonvulsant compounds) and radiation (including sunlight).

Most human autoimmune diseases are much more common in women than in men. It has also been observed that a number of different autoimmune diseases tend to cluster in members of some families. Why this should be so is not yet understood.

It is interesting to speculate why more women suffer from autoimmune diseases than men. As we saw in Chapter 4, immune functioning is influenced by emotional and psychological processes, and people with autoimmune diseases seem to show a pronounced tendency to repress anger and other negative emotions. Traditionally it has been women in our society who have been discouraged from expressing anger, and this may help to account for the high incidence of autoimmune diseases in women.

Whatever the specific cause, autoimmune diseases are on the increase today. The stresses of daily life, combined with the unresolved role conflicts that both women and men experience, may well help to account for the unfortunate "boom" in this important category of illness.

We will begin our review of some representative autoimmune diseases by discussing some familiar and common ones, and then touch on a few that are less well known.

RHEUMATOID ARTHRITIS

Probably the most familiar of the autoimmune diseases is rheumatoid arthritis, or RA. One to 3 percent of Americans have RA, with women three times more likely than men to develop the disease. The onset of RA typically occurs between the ages of twenty-five and fifty, but it can attack at any age. It is not unusual to see children with RA moving with painful stiffness like elderly arthritics.

The disease is characterized by a chronic inflammation of the synovium, the thin membrane that surrounds a joint. Gradually the inflammation spreads to other parts of the joint, with a build-up of lymphoid cells, resulting in degeneration of cartilage, bone, ligaments, and tendons. The damaged joint is then subject to dislocation, instability, loss of range of motion, stiffness, deformity, and severe pain. The pain and stiffness are worse after resting and gradually diminish with activity.

Rheumatoid arthritis is not just a disease of the joints, but of the whole body. It can cause a generalized inflammation of the heart, blood vessels, and tissues beneath the skin, and fibrous deposits in the lungs.

According to one theory, rheumatoid arthritis may begin with joint inflammation caused by an infectious agent — perhaps the Epstein-Barr virus, which causes infectious mononucleosis. Antibodies produced in response to this inflammation may be damaged by enzymes and then be perceived as foreign antigens by the immune system. These are then attacked by other antibodies, including the so-called rheumatoid factor, bringing about the typical degenerative changes of RA.

On the assumption that autoimmunity is involved in rheumatoid arthritis, the disease is sometimes treated with immunosuppressive drugs or radiation. Such measures are quite drastic, since they weaken the body's defenses against infection and cancer.

According to some clinicians, rheumatoid arthritis may be *many* diseases, not one. Clinically there are two distinct manifestations of this disease — the *highly episodic* form (very bad one day, followed by remission, then very bad again, days later, and so on) and a *slowly progressive* form (not better or worse from day to day, just slowly getting worse).

The therapy discussed below is particularly useful in the episodic form of the disease.

A protozoal connection in RA? A disease as poorly understood as rheumatoid arthritis may require a multifaceted approach. In this light, it is reasonable to mention the work of Roger Wyburn-Mason, M.D., a brilliant English physician. His discoveries about the cause and treatment of this ravaging disease have been neglected or shunned in his home country, but a Japanese publisher wisely brought out the large volume of Dr. Wyburn-Mason's work in 1978.

This remarkable book, based on hundreds of cases, argues that we are all parasitized by amoebas and suggests that these may be the *causative agents* in rheumatoid arthritis. Dr. Wyburn-Mason makes a strong, convincing argument for the use of clotrimazole (not available in the United States), a classic antimalarial drug, for treating RA. In America, the drug Flagelle is used for this purpose by interested physicians. Experience with hundreds of RA patients has shown an 80 percent rate of remission with use of this drug,* which is normally prescribed to destroy amoebas in certain vaginal infections.

Remember to advise your physician, if you undertake this therapy, to expect a *Herxheimer's reaction.* This means that you may get worse before you get better on this treatment, because as the amoebas are killed (assuming they *are* present), they release toxins that are more damaging to the system than are live amoebas.

Dr. Wyburn-Mason's theories may not apply to all cases of RA, but his suggested treatment regimen deserves exploration by any sincere physician.

As a final caution for RA sufferers, two British doctors have

---

*For complete details, you may want to contact Jack M. Blount, M.D., director, Rheumatoid Disease Foundation, Route 4, Box 137, Franklin, TN 37064.

suggested that excess iron in the system can accumulate in the synovial membranes and attract immune cells that release substances that interact with the iron to produce damaging hydroxyl radicals. It is the hydroxyl radical, they suggest, that produces the pain, swelling, and synovial damage in RA. Iron-deficient populations rarely are bothered by this disease (Martin 1984). Perhaps RA patients would do well to limit their use of iron supplements.

SYSTEMIC LUPUS ERYTHEMATOSUS

Systemic lupus erythematosus, or SLE, is a stereotypic autoimmune disease, with antibodies in the blood attacking almost every possible kind of tissue. Antigen-antibody complexes accumulate throughout the body and are destroyed along with surrounding tissues, as well as interfering with normal organ functions. As a result, there can be damage to the joints, lymph nodes, spleen, liver, lungs, and gastrointestinal tract, and internal bleeding of the kidneys and heart.

A characteristic symptom of the disease is a red, butterfly-shaped rash across the bridge of the nose and the upper cheeks. (The name of the disease means "red wolf.") Most SLE patients have arthritic joint pain and swelling, and kidney problems. Less frequently the central nervous system is affected, with epileptic seizures, psychotic symptoms, or personality changes. Other problems may include fatigue, fever, chills, and headache. Many lupus victims lose their hair, but it usually grows back rapidly. In the past, kidney disease was responsible for a high mortality rate among SLE victims. Today, with improved diagnosis and early therapy, progressive kidney disease usually can be prevented.

Lupus is a chronic and lifelong disorder, but with proper treatment need not be life threatening. Because its symptoms imitate a variety of other diseases, lupus was not always properly diagnosed in the past. Today it is known to be much more common than was previously thought. As many as one million Americans have lupus, of whom *80 to 90 percent are women,* most of them between twenty and forty. There is also some evidence that blacks may be more affected than whites.

Treatment for lupus depends on the severity of the disease.

Anti-inflammatory drugs, ranging from aspirin to corticosteroids, help to control most of the symptoms.

DIABETES MELLITUS

Diabetes, including its complications, is the third most common cause of death in the United States, after heart disease and cancer. It may surprise you to learn that one form of this widespread disease is believed to be autoimmune in nature.

There are two main types of diabetes. Type I is known as insulin dependent diabetes mellitus, or IDDM; formerly it was called juvenile-onset diabetes because it generally appears during youth. Type II diabetes is known today as non-insulin-dependent diabetes mellitus, or NIDDM. It has also been called maturity-onset diabetes, or obesity-induced diabetes mellitus. It is Type I, or IDDM, that is suspected to be an autoimmune disorder. Type II is generally much less serious and can usually be managed by diet, exercise, and if necessary, oral medications, while IDDM generally requires injections of insulin throughout the patient's lifetime.

Of the approximately 11 million Americans with diabetes, some 1.5 million suffer from IDDM. The average age of onset is about twelve; by the age of eighteen, one out of every 300 to 400 Caucasian youths in the United States has developed the disease. Whereas Type II diabetes is generally slow to develop, IDDM is usually relatively abrupt in its onset. There seems to be a genetic component in diabetes. People with a family history of the disease have about twenty-five times greater chance of developing the disease than those from unaffected families.

IDDM is characterized by the progressive destruction of the beta cells, which are responsible for producing the hormone insulin, in the islets of Langerhans in the pancreas. Without insulin to regulate blood sugar, the body suffers a number of harmful effects. The excess sugar in the blood causes excessive loss of fluids and minerals, with possible dehydration or kidney damage. Without enough insulin, the muscles burn fat instead of sugar, and the resultant fatty acid residues can produce atherosclerotic deposits in the arteries. Thus diabetics are at a much higher than average risk of developing blood vessel and heart disease.

The burning of fats also leads to elevated levels of ketones in the blood, producing a condition known as acidosis, which can result in diabetic coma, in which the victim can lose consciousness and may even die. IDDM can also produce neuropathy, or nerve damage, which can lead to blindness and insensitivity to pain.

To prevent all of these dangerous complications, the IDDM patient must usually follow a lifelong program of blood glucose testing and self-administered insulin injections to keep blood sugar within safe limits.

IDDM has several characteristics of an autoimmune disease, including the presence of antibodies that attack the beta cells of the pancreas. These anti-beta cell antibodies appear in the individual's blood before actual symptoms of IDDM develop (Forsham et al. 1983; Cahill and McDevitt 1981). Another sign of autoimmune mechanisms in IDDM is elevated levels of T cells bearing the Ia (immune-associated) antigen. Such Ia-bearing T cells are also elevated in people with other autoimmune disorders, such as rheumatoid arthritis and systemic lupus erythematosus (Jackson et al. 1982).

Animal studies also bear out the role of autoimmunity in IDDM. Using a strain of rats with a genetic predisposition toward diabetes, researchers prevented some of these rats from developing IDDM by blocking their immune system (Rossini 1983). While immunosuppressive drugs have been used experimentally to treat IDDM, we know that suppressing the immune system leaves the individual open to attack from a wide range of pathogens and also possibly to the increased likelihood of cancer.

SCLERODERMA

Another autoimmune disease of unknown cause, scleroderma (literally, "hard skin"), affects at least three hundred thousand people in the United States. It is rare among people under twenty and affects more women than men. The disease takes two forms. *Localized* scleroderma affects the skin and subcutaneous tissues, creating cosmetic disfigurement and difficult mobility. *Systemic* scleroderma is much more serious, affecting the internal organs, including the esophagus, heart, lungs, intestines, and kidneys, as well as skin areas. The five-year survival rate for this form of the disease is less than 50 percent, with the most common cause of death being cardiopulmonary disease and kidney failure.

Scleroderma usually appears first in the hands and/or feet, with the skin becoming thick, tight, and hard. An early indicator of the disease is often *Raynaud's phenomenon,* a disturbance of the blood vessels in the extremities. Circulation becomes impaired, especially on exposure to cold. The hands may change color from white to blue to red, with pain, tingling, numbness, or burning. The circulation problem can result in the loss or atrophy of fingers or toes. (Note that Raynaud's *alone* is not a sure sign of scleroderma. Raynaud's usually occurs without the presence of another disease.)

In the systemic form of the disease, gastrointestinal problems are common. Seventy-five percent of scleroderma patients have problems with the esophagus, including difficulty swallowing, heartburn, esophageal scarring from acid reflux, and a bitter taste. The small intestine may also be affected, with diarrhea and gas. Practically all scleroderma patients also develop lung problems (Diamond 1982).

The autoimmune components of scleroderma include the presence of antinuclear antibodies and rheumatoid factor, and the local infiltration of white cells in the affected tissues. There is no known treatment for this very serious disease. In the future an immunosuppressive approach, despite the risks of such a drastic form of therapy, may be developed.

MYASTHENIA GRAVIS

This disease may affect as many as one hundred thousand people in the United States. Although it can strike anyone at any age, symptoms generally appear earlier in females (most commonly between fifteen and thirty-five) than in males (usually between forty and seventy).

Myasthenia gravis is a chronic neuromuscular disease marked by weakness and abnormally rapid fatigue of the voluntary muscles. The symptoms improve with rest. The muscles most commonly affected are those around the eyes and those used for swallowing.

The disease appears to be associated with tumor or other abnormalities of the thymus and with the production of an antibody that attacks striated (voluntary) muscle tissue. Removal of the thymus has produced remissions ranging from 25 to 75 percent and is considered especially beneficial in young women. Corticosteroids and anticholinesterase drugs are also used to treat the symptoms. Myasthenia gravis is considered one of the most successfully managed of the neurological disorders.

RHEUMATIC FEVER

Rheumatic fever involves the development of an autoimmune response to heart tissue, typically following repeated streptococcal infections of the mouth and throat. It usually occurs between the ages of five and fifteen. Symptoms of the disease include fever, sore and swollen joints, skin rash, and involuntary muscle twitching. The heart valves may become scarred and unable to close completely, interfering with the proper flow of blood through the heart. Heart murmurs may result. Antibiotics are often given following rheumatic fever to prevent recurrence of the disease or further damage to the heart.

ASPERMATOGENESIS

In this condition, a man produces antibodies against his own sperm, causing the sperm to clump together or become immobilized. In about 2 to 3 percent of infertile couples, the problem has been traced to aspermatogenesis in the male partner.

Since sperm do not develop until puberty, long after the immune system has become established, it is not surprising that they can serve as autoantigens. When the sperm appear, they may provoke an immune response, leaving the male effectively infertile.

A WIDE VARIETY OF DISEASES
ARE AUTOIMMUNE

In this chapter, we have described only a few of the autoimmune diseases. Table 15 lists a wide variety of troublesome diseases in which autoimmune mechanisms are presently established or suspected. If autoimmune diseases are increasing in prevalence, and

TABLE 15

Some Human Diseases
with Autoimmune Manifestations

Disease	Antigen (Body Part Attacked)
Endocrine	
Chronic thyroiditis (Hashimoto's disease) and primary myxedema	Thyroglobulin Microsomes Membranous portion of microsomes
Adrenal insufficiency (Addison's disease)	Microsomes of adrenal cortex Steroid-producing cells
Primary hypopituitarism	Anterior pituitary
Primary hypoparathyroidism	Oxyphilic cells Principal cells
Gastrointestinal	
Pernicious anemia (Addisonian) and atrophic gastritis	Intrinsic factor Parietal cells
Ulcerative colitis	Colonic mucosal cells *Escherichia coli*
Primary biliary cirrhosis	Mitochondria
Reproductive	
Orchitis and masculine sterility	Spermatozoa Germinal epithelium
Eye	
Endophthalmitis phacoanaphylactic	Lens
Sympathetic ophthalmia	Uvea
Neurologic	
Postvaccinal encephalitis and postinfectious encephalitis	Myelin or basic protein of brain or spinal cord
Polyneuritis and neuropathy (Guillain-Barré syndrome)	Peripheral nervous tissue
Heart and Kidney	
Postcardiotomy syndrome	Cardiac muscle
Postinfarction syndrome of Dressler	Cardiac muscle
Rheumatic fever	Subsarcolemmal membrane of cardiac muscle Group A streptococcal cell surface
Autoimmune glomerulonephritis (Goodpasture's syndrome)	Glomerular basement membrane of the kidney Septal alveolar membranes of lung
Immune complex glomerulonephritis	Tubular epithelium and brush border of kidney or nuclear components

Disease	Antigen (Body Part Attacked)
Connective Tissue	
Systemic lupus erythematosus	Nuclear components Mitochondria
Rheumatoid arthritis	Denatured IgG Collagen Epstein-Barr related antigens
Scleroderma	Nuclear components Collagen
Polymyositis and dermatomyositis	Nuclear components Collagen
Neuromuscular	
Myasthenia gravis	Striations of skeletal and cardiac muscle (acetylcholine receptors)
Exocrine Glands	
Keratoconjunctivitis sicca (Sjögren's disease)	Salivary gland
Skin	
Pemphigus vulgaris	Intercellular substance of skin and mucosa
Bullous pemphigoid	Basal membrane of skin and mucosa
Blood	
Acquired hemolytic anemia	Red blood cells
Idiopathic thrombocytopenic purpura	Platelets
Leukopenia	Leukocytes

Source: Rose, Milgrom, and van Oss, 1976

if environmental factors do play a role, then the best protection against them is to bolster your immune defenses. A proper diet, supplying all the protective nutrients, and a healthy, positive attitude, supported by adequate stress management and stimulated by exercise, may help you to evade this mysterious group of diseases in which self literally attacks self.

HOW DO WE KNOW IF DIET, ATTITUDE, AND EXERCISE WILL ACTUALLY PROTECT US?

The fact is we do not have definite proof in the form of solid, scientific studies that diet, exercise, and attitude will actually protect us. But the evidence is very strong that we can stimulate our own internal pharmacopoeia to defeat whatever may be bringing on these diseases. While we can say only that the techniques of immune stimulation suggested here "may help" protect against these diseases, or even reverse them, in some cases, this "may" is based on the best available information.

We have seen how negative emotions caused by grief, despair, or chronic depression depress the T and B cells in our immune system. If such emotions can bring about immune suppression, then the reverse must also be true. Positive emotions should be able to prevent immune-related disorders or help conquer them should they occur. The same line of experience with nutrients and physical activity leads us to believe that these, too, can help prevent or reverse such illnesses. All the evidence is not yet in, but we know enough to trust our own powers of healing, as augmented by the parameters of immune stimulation.

As the writer Norman Cousins said in a recent interview, "I see a time coming in the development of medicine when doctors will continue to prescribe, but their prescriptions will not be on the basis of what they can put into the body, but on what they can get the body to do" (*New Realities*, February 1985).

○ 12 ○

Immune Deficiency Diseases

"IMMUNE DEFICIENCY" has become something of a buzz term now that the AIDS epidemic has made us so acutely aware of the importance of our immune defenses. But AIDS is only one of a wide variety of immune deficiency diseases, some of them genetic and some acquired later in life.

Earlier we presented the story of David, the boy who had to live in a hermetically sealed, germ-free environment because his immune system was unable to fight off disease. We also hear from time to time about transplant patients who succumb to pneumonia or cancer because their immune systems have been suppressed by drugs to prevent rejection. The American public is further haunted by the image of millions of starving children worldwide, whose severe malnutrition reduces their immune functioning and exposes them to a greatly increased risk of infection. All of these problems are examples of immune deficiencies. In severe cases, both genetic and acquired immunodeficiencies can leave the victim helplessly exposed to a barrage of pathogens that would be harmless to people with normal immune systems.

In all the various immune deficiency disorders, the lymphocytes or the antibodies produced by the B cells, or both, are either absent or insufficient. The problem may arise in the stem cells in the bone marrow, from which the white blood cells are formed; in the parts of the body where the white blood cells mature and differentiate; or in the final balance of the various cells needed to regulate immune functioning (Cunningham 1978). As we have seen throughout the book, a wide variety of factors can inhibit white blood cell production and function, including faulty genes, drugs, radiation, surgery, traumatic injury, malnutrition, stress, or hormonal imbalances. These health-destroying factors should be evaluated — and avoided when possible — in trying to determine how the following diseases come about.

PRIMARY IMMUNODEFICIENCY DISEASES

Many of the immune deficiency disorders that affect infants are due to faulty genes. However, such primary immune deficiencies may not show up until later in life, depending on the severity of the immune disorder and the degree of exposure to antigens.

The role of genetics in these immune deficiency diseases was not fully recognized until the 1950s; before then they were classified as "congenital" or "acquired," depending on when symptoms began to appear.

Some genetic immune deficiencies are due to a defect in the autosomal (nonsex) genes, while in others the genetic defect is in a sex-linked recessive gene. In the latter case, the mother is usually a *carrier* of the defective gene, but does not herself show the immune deficiency. The gene is passed on to roughly half her offspring. When it is passed on to a daughter, she too becomes a carrier, while a son who inherits the gene will be affected by the immune deficiency. The defective gene may remain hidden in the female carriers for generations before finally showing itself in an affected male. A female can be affected by this particular kind of deficiency only if both her mother and father passed the faulty gene on to her.

The primary immune deficiency diseases are classified according to which parts of the immune system they affect: *thymus related,* or those in which the T cells (cellular immunity) are impaired; *antibody related,* in which the B cells (humoral immunity) are impaired; and a *combination* of cellular and humoral immunity impairments.

DiGeorge syndrome. This primary immune deficiency disease involves an impairment of cellular immunity (thymus and T cells). B cell function and antibody levels are usually normal. Because the production of T cells is depressed, the person with Di-George syndrome is highly susceptible to viral and fungal infections (which are combated by the T cells). Death usually occurs before the age of two. In a few cases, T cell function has been restored for a few years by implanting the thymus gland from a human fetus (Rose, Milgrom, and van Oss 1976).

Bruton's syndrome. This disease is caused by a sex-linked recessive gene. Bruton's involves failure of humoral immunity, or the production of antibodies by the B cells. The thymus-dependent system functions normally. Since the antibodies fight bacteria, people with Bruton's syndrome are highly susceptible to bacterial infection, while they have normal resistance to viruses. Such common viral infections as smallpox, measles, and mumps are no more of a problem to a B deficient individual than they are to one who is immunocompetent.

Symptoms of Bruton's syndrome generally do not appear until about six months after birth, since up to that time the infant is protected by antibodies acquired from the mother. Some people with Bruton's are never able to produce detectable amounts of antibody, but periodic antibody injections keep this disease from being fatal.

Swiss type agammaglobulinemia. This disease is an example of an impairment of both humoral and cellular immunity. Swiss-type disease is a very serious *severe combined immunodeficiency* (SCID), with both T cell and antibody-dependent systems completely absent. Infants with this disorder usually die during their first two years from massive infections of all types — bacterial, viral, and fungal. David, the "bubble boy," was a victim of SCID. The only hope for children with this disorder is a bone marrow transplant from a closely related donor. Such transplants, usually from siblings, have saved the lives of some SCID youngsters. In David's case, as we have mentioned, the bone marrow transplant did not take, and he died of complications of his disease.

SECONDARY IMMUNE DEFICIENCY DISEASES

As we have already seen, not all immune deficiencies are genetic in origin. Immune deficiencies may develop at any time in the life cycle as a result of nongenetic factors, including aging, stress, malnutrition, immunosuppressants such as drugs or radiation, certain disease states, ór malignancies. Such influences can cause one or more components of the immune system to shut down.

Of the secondary immune deficiency diseases, by far the most publicity has been given to AIDS. This mysterious and disturbing complex of at least two dozen different "opportunistic" infections is such a large subject that it has been treated separately in Chapter 10.

A characteristic of AIDS is an imbalance between the T helper and suppressor cells. Such imbalances between the various components of the immune system are probably responsible for many of the immune deficiency diseases that develop later in life. As in the case of AIDS, these imbalances may be caused by a complex combination of factors that may stimulate or suppress the immune response.

Immunosuppressants. In Chapter 9, in our discussion of cancer, we mentioned that many agents, from both within and outside the body, can suppress immune functioning. Radiation, whether used therapeutically or emanated from a nuclear waste site, can suppress the immune response and perhaps lead to cancer. Even sunlight can be a threat to your bodily defenses; as we learned, excessive exposure to sunlight can lead to melanoma.

We will now review some of the other agents that can depress immunity and lead to the development of secondary immune deficiency diseases.

Corticosteroids are the hormones produced in the adrenal cortex. They include cortisol, corticosterone, aldosterone, cortisone, and other natural hormones, as well as synthetically produced ones. These hormones are often used to control allergic reactions, and they are used as anti-inflammatory agents in organ transplants, to prevent graft rejection. The corticosteroids act as immunosuppressants, reducing the size and contents of the lymph nodes and interfering with phagocytosis. As we discussed in Chapter 4, stress has been shown to cause an increase in corticosteroid levels in the system, which helps to explain how stress can suppress immune function.

Cytotoxic chemicals are chemicals that are harmful to the cells. This fascinating group of substances, while having obvious immunosuppressive effects as well as the ability to kill cells, ironically has important applications in medicine. The *alkylating agents,* for example, include the so-called nitrogen mustards and others. Originally developed as agents for chemical warfare, they are used today in cancer chemotherapy. One of the nitrogen mustards, cyclophosphamide, is also used to prevent graft rejection. The *antimetabolites* are protein synthesis inhibitors (remember that antibody is a protein). Fluorouracil, for example, is used in cancer of the breast, colon, and other organs, and mercaptopurine is used in the leukemias. Another antimetabolite, azathioprine, is very commonly used to help suppress rejection of grafts. The antimetabolite methotrexate seems to inhibit lymphocyte proliferation; it is used to treat a variety of cancers and, less commonly, to act as an immunosuppressant in transplant cases.

Although they are used widely in medicine today, these cytotoxic chemicals can produce very serious complications, including increased susceptibility to infection, possible genetic damage, and increased risk of cancer. It is hoped that other substances may be available in the future, perhaps based on derivatives of natural plant sources, that will be able to help cancer patients without the disturbing side effects of these drugs.

Environmental pollutants are becoming an increased cause of concern as a source of immunosuppression. Many *pesticides,* for example, have been banned from use on crops in the United States because they have been shown to cause cancer, birth defects, and other serious problems in laboratory animals. Organochlorine pesticides (including DDT, lindane, dieldrin, and chlordane) have been sharply curtailed by the EPA, and so today most pesticides used are organophosphates or carbamates — substances that break down fairly rapidly (unlike the organochlorine pesticides), reducing the risk of cumulative damage. However, in large doses the organophosphates and carbamates may cause serious nervous system disorders, and thousands of agricultural and chemical workers are poisoned by them every year.

Many pesticides have been shown to affect the immune defenses of animals, and in some cases of humans. Pesticides have also been associated with allergic responses, and in some cases certain pesticides have been linked with autoimmune diseases (Sharma 1981).

As long as our produce is being sprayed, we strongly recommend that you wash your fruits and vegetables thoroughly, removing all outer layers whenever possible.

Other environmental pollutants get into the food chain, our water supply, and our atmosphere through industrial processes, chemical dumping, and other means peculiar to our modern industrial world. Chemicals such as methylmercury chloride, mercury chloride, cobalt sulfate, nickel acetate, and disodium chromate have been shown to suppress immunological reactions and increase susceptibility to viral infection in test animals (Sharma 1981). Also, lead, cadmium, mercury, methylmercury, nickel, cobalt, chromium, and platinum reduce antibody levels against specific antigens, while selenium, copper, and manganese increase some antibody levels (Sharma 1981).

Arsenic-containing compounds also increase susceptibility to viral infection, by depressing the immune response and by interfering with interferon, a protein that occurs naturally in cells and is very effective in battling viruses.

Other immunosuppressive agents, in addition to the above, may include stress, malnutrition, viruses, bacteria, alcohol, and allergens. The degree to which they suppress the immune system depends upon their intensity and the underlying state of the host's immune system. This means, once again, that your best protection against these environmental immunosuppressants is a combination of proper diet, stress management and a positive psychological outlook, and exercise.

In addition to the factors already mentioned, you will also want to look at the kinds of "quiet stresses" that we sometimes bring onto ourselves; such stresses can result in illness. Serious and chronic dieting can deprive us of essential, protective nutrients. Too many x rays, or too frequent air travel with inadequate rest, are other silent immune depressants. Chronic, untreated depression, or too many surgical procedures can also bring about lowered immunity, which raises the risk of diseases. While proof positive showing the above relationships does not yet exist, as with the autoimmune diseases, we have the vectors of information necessary to act. A conscious will to heal ourselves, or protect ourselves against these or other diseases, sets up the internal defenses needed to do the work.

∘ 13 ∘

Candidiasis

OR THE BEASTLY YEAST

IN SOME CIRCLES of alternative medicine, candidiasis is now seen as the disease underlying a wide range of complaints, much as hypoglycemia, or low-blood sugar, was the "fad" disease of the 1970s. While thousands, perhaps hundreds of thousands, of genuine cases of candidiasis can and will be verified, we *can not* look to this disease as the mother of all complaints and to its eradication as a panacea for all attendant ills.

Nevertheless, a number of reputable clinicians are convinced of the seriousness of this illness, and it has appeared in a great enough number of people to warrant a chapter. In addition, a conference of physicians and scientists devoted exclusively to "The Yeast-Human Interaction" was held in San Francisco during March 1985.

This fungal disease is spreading rapidly, especially among women in the United States. It is clearly a disease related to depressed immune functioning and often responds to immune-enhancing intervention.

Caused by the yeastlike organism *Candida albicans,* candidiasis generally infects the skin, nails, mouth, vagina, bronchi, or lungs but can invade the blood stream as well.

When it infects the mouth, as oral candidiasis, it is commonly known as *thrush.* This used to be found most often in newborn infants, who became infected as they passed through the vagina, where the fungus is found in a great percentage of women. A cream-colored or gray, loose membrane appears, which is painful and bleeds easily. This infection is also a problem in older people as a result of suppressed resistance.

What is especially alarming is the recent report that a high percentage of patients diagnosed as having AIDS have previously had chronic thrush. Even more disturbing is the observation of AIDS in twenty-three African patients, living in Belgium, with *no* history of homosexuality, blood product transfusion, intravenous drug abuse, or an underlying disease that suppresses the immune system (Clumeck et al. 1984). But eight of fifteen patients in one group of the twenty-three studied were diagnosed as having various opportunistic infections, including chronic *Candida albicans!* In some patients this "simple thrush" had become invasive, spreading to the esophagus, lungs, or stomach.

The threat of this once mildly viewed disease is not limited to our fear that it can invade the deep tissues and produce fatal illness. Even in its less virulent form (clinically exemplified by white patches on the tongue), this ubiquitous fungus often causes clinical symptoms that are very difficult to live with.

WHAT CAUSES THIS INFECTION?

It seems that antibiotic therapy often leads to a killing of microbes that keep candida in a state of balance with other "normal" microflora. In such circumstances, or as a result of a disease that diminishes immune competence, the normal candida population goes through abnormal growth, leading to the "yeast infection" millions of women have learned to live with.

Other, *indirect* methods of ingestion of antibiotics, such as from meat, may also explain this new epidemic. Oral contraceptives are another factor, because they can directly stimulate the growth of candida. An altered acid/alkaline balance (pH) in the gut (due to faulty diet) also creates a good growing medium for this invasive microbe.

THE NATURAL HISTORY

Candida can produce a wide range of symptoms that may be mistaken for other illnesses. A leading biochemist, Jeffrey Bland, Ph.D., in an article in *Preventive Medicine,* summarizes some of the deceptive symptoms that have been traced to candida infection.

Patients may have heard many times from doctors that they are suffering from "neurotic anxiety syndrome" when they complain of depression, anxiety, recurring irritability, heartburn, indigestion, lethargy, extreme food and environmental allergies, acne, migraine headaches, recurring cystitis or vaginal infections, premenstrual tension or menstrual problems, all of which have not been identified with any disease entity.... The explanation is locked into understanding the life cycle of a symbiotic yeast become a parasite called *Candida albicans*. (Bland 1984)

Dr. Bland credits Dr. C. Orian Truss of Birmingham, Alabama, for doing the pioneering work in understanding the role of candida in this symptom complex.

Present in everyone from early infancy, this yeastlike organism lives in the intestinal tract, usually without producing overt symptoms. During periods of stress, or when the immune system is otherwise suppressed, the candida organism can increase in numbers. Here is where the long-term use of antibiotics or of oral contraceptives can trigger candida overgrowth. What can happen next is described by Dr. Bland in disturbing detail.

As *Candida* proliferates in the intestines, it can change its anatomy and physiology from the yeast-like form to the mycelial fungal form. It is well recognized that *Candida albicans* is a dimorphic organism and as such can exist in these two states. The yeast-like state is a non-invasive, sugar-fermenting organism, whereas the fungal state produces rhizoids, or very long root-like structures, which can penetrate the mucosa, and it is invasive. Penetration of the gastrointestinal mucosa can break down the boundary between the intestinal tract and the rest of the circulation and allow introduction into the blood stream of many substances which may be antigenic. Such things as incompletely digested dietary proteins may be delivered to the blood through the portals of entry of the intestinal tract produced by the invasive mycelia of the fungal form of *Candida albicans*. This may explain why many individuals who have chronic *Candida* overgrowth and a high percentage of the mycelial form of the organism commonly show a wide variety of food and environmental allergies. These incompletely digested dietary proteins can then travel into the blood stream and exert a powerful antigenic assault on the immune system, which is seen as allergy, even producing a wide variety of effects such as cerebral allergy, with depression, mood swings and irritability being a result. . . .

The breakdown of the gastrointestinal mucosa can also lead to the introduction of the *Candida* organism into the blood stream and it can then find its way into other tissues, resulting in far-ranging systemic effects, including soreness of joints, chest pain and skin problems.

One of the common side effects of chronic *Candida* infection is recurring vaginal infections or cystitis. We all harbor the organism in our bodies, but it is when the body loses its proper immune protection, or the intestinal pH is altered unfavorably, that the organism can then proliferate and change its state from the yeast form to the fungal form. (Bland 1984)

AN ALTERNATIVE TREATMENT PROGRAM

The yeast form of *Candida albicans* is much easier to treat than the fungal form. One of the aims of treatment, therefore, is to prevent the yeast from converting to the fungal form. Antiyeast medications such as nystatin may need to be continued for six to nine months before symptoms are relieved.

An alternative approach to candidiasis which does not involve the antiyeast medication has been used with some success. Dr. Bland describes this program as follows:

1. *Reinoculate bowel.* It is well recognized that a disturbed flora of the gastrointestinal tract can establish a proper environment for the yeast proliferation. By reinoculating the bowel with proper symbiotic acid-producing bacteria, there is a reduction in the compatibility of the intestinal environment for yeast proliferation. We have recently used an oral supplement of *Lactobacillus acidophilus,* cultured from mother's milk, to reinoculate the bowel. This has been extremely successful in reducing *Candida albicans* in the intestinal tract. The *Lactobacillus acidophilus* mixture is given as a dry culture (1 teaspoon taken three times daily).

2. *Prevent conversion.* The second portion of the program, which is extremely important, is the recognition that the conversion of the yeast form to the fungal form of *Candida* is partially dependent upon biotin deficiency. . . . When biotin is added to the medium in high levels, it can prevent the conversion of the yeast form of *Candida* to its fungal form. . . . The fatty acid *oleic acid* also seems to prevent this same conversion.

This concept has been used very successfully in conjunction

with the *Lactobacillus acidophilus* culture to treat *Candida albicans.*
Biotin is given orally (300 mcg taken three times daily) along
with two teaspoons of *olive oil* taken three times daily, as a source
of oleic acid. This is done along with a higher than normal fiber
diet, using *oat bran fiber,* to increase the absorptive surface area of
the fecal material and to hasten the elimination of metabolic
by-products. This may have to be continued for a period of one
to six months depending upon the severity of the infection and
the length of time that there has been a *Candida* problem.

3. *Heal GI mucosa.* Once the organism is arrested in its growth and
has been converted back to the yeast form, a program is then
instituted to facilitate the healing of the gastrointestinal mucosa. This program includes higher levels of *zinc* (30 to 50 mg a
day), *vitamin E* (400 to 800 I.U. per day), and *calcium pentothenate*
(200 to 1000 mg per day). (Bland 1984)

On this program, there should be an improvement of symptoms,
which may range from multiple allergies and headaches to skin
problems or menstrual irregularities. Dr. Bland reports that the
program has been helpful in more than 50 percent of the patients
who have used it to alleviate chronic problems that were otherwise hard to diagnose and apparently untreatable. He reports
that "cases such as 10- to 15-year recurrent migraine headaches
have been alleviated by the use of this program, as well as long-
standing adult acne and joint pain resembling arthritis, which
may really be a result of the buildup of immunochemically reactive materials from the direct or indirect effects of *Candida*"
(Bland 1984).

While not everyone with fatigue, mood swings, headaches, or
other central nervous system problems is suffering from candidiasis, this problem is widespread and should be considered in
people with intractable, recurring symptoms of this kind. The
treatment program outlined above provides a viable alternative
to synthetic antifungal medications and will help restore normal
bowel flora and, it is hoped, rebalance immune function.

OTHER TREATMENTS

Numerous recent symposiums and publications, both by the medical community and former sufferers from this condition, attest to

other treatments with high rates of success. Classic double-blind studies have not yet confirmed or denied these reports, but we must trust the observations of skilled clinicians.

Even skeptical physicians will acknowledge that there *is* a condition known as candidiasis, depending upon a demonstration of *Candida albicans* overgrowth or tissue invasion. What we are talking about in this chapter may be termed "atypical" candidiasis, which is a term for several syndromes that show clinical improvement following the use of specific antifungal medications along with a variety of environmental and dietary modifications specially designed for their "anticandida" effects.

The first drug generally used is the "standard," nystatin. But there are several disadvantages to using this powerful pharmaceutical, including the fact that it is *not* a broad-spectrum killer of fungi and may miss the target organisms causing this syndrome. Several strains of candida resistant to nystatin have been described. And, as with antibiotics, an increased use of this drug might lead to the emergence of organisms resistant to nystatin. This and other problems with nystatin have led to the development of other treatments.

Two products receiving wide reports of success with safety (Da Prato pers. com. 1984; 1985) are based on their immunological properties. The apparent immune tolerance and bizarre reactions to foods and chemicals seen in atypical candidiasis may be due in part to depression of enzyme function. By removing the disease organism at the site of entry, normal function is seen to return. Nutrient-based products that control the overgrowth of yeast, both systemically as well as in the mouth and vagina, would logically enhance immunity. One of these products is composed of a fatty acid (caprylic acid, a derivative of coconut oil) that exhibits fungicidal action, most specifically against *Candida albicans* (Da Prato 1984). This nutritional product, known as Caprystatin, was tested clinically in an earlier form at the University of Illinois College of Medicine. "All patients showed complete disappearance of Candida from stool specimens in several days . . . these patients experienced a remission of symptoms associated with systemic Candidiasis" (Neuhauser and Gustus 1954).

As early as 1946, caprylic acid was used in the treatment of chronic yeast infections. In 1954 Irene Neuhauser, M.D., associate clinical professor of dermatology at the University of Illinois College of Medicine, reported on the successful use of a caprylic acid complex for patients with severe candidiasis. Most of the patients studied at the university had suffered a long-standing yeast infection that had been resistant to treatment by traditional antifungal medications. Following two months of treatment with this caprylic acid complex, most patients experienced a complete remission of symptoms. While this noteworthy study was published in the AMA journal, *Archives of Internal Medicine,* it was overshadowed by the rash of articles on antibiotics for the next thirty years. As antibiotics came to the fore and were widely prescribed for nonspecific ailments, chronic candidiasis became a rapidly growing problem.

Recently, Ecological Formulas, of Concord, California, has introduced a nonallergenic caprylic acid product, similar to the one used by Dr. Neuhauser in the treatment of candidiasis. This nutritional supplement, Caprystatin,* has been used successfully for resistant yeast infections and is available without a prescription. Many prominent physicians who have used it in their treatment regimen have found that its effectiveness exceeds that of nystatin. It is important that caprylic acid is released slowly to coat the broadest possible surface area of the intestines. Once the yeast infection in the lower bowel is controlled, other infections in the mouth, esophagus, bladder, and vagina will clear up more rapidly.

To facilitate control of oral and vaginal yeast overgrowth, another fatty acid is used in a topical preparation. Sorbic acid, a fatty acid derived from the berries of mountain ash, is one of the most effective and rapid-acting treatments for candidiasis in mucocutaneous regions. Orithrush Gargle and Mouth Rinse and Orithrush Douche Concentrate are two companion products for candidiasis supplied by Ecological Formulas. The original use of a buffered form of sorbic acid was studied by two gynecologists, E. Rodgerson and D. McKinnon, who reported their findings in the

*Caprystatin and Orithrush are registered trademarks of Ecological Formulas. Further information on the nutritional management of candida may be obtained by writing to Ecological Formulas, 1061-B Shary Circle, Concord, CA 94518; or calling (415) 827-2636.

journal *Obstetrics and Gynecology* (1973). More than 80 percent of the patients with yeast vaginitis who were treated with sorbic acid experienced rapid relief within twenty-four hours of application.

The ideal program for self-recovery from yeast infections incorporates a low-carbohydrate, low-yeast diet along with the introduction of Pau D'Arco tea, caprylic acid, sorbic acid, and other accessory nutrient factors. Avoidance of certain stressors and medications will hasten the road to recovery.

HERBAL TEAS AGAINST YEAST

The biggest "underground" news in successfully controlling candidiasis comes from the world of healing plants. Good results with a tea from South America have been reported by many physicians, including Phyllis Saifer, M.D., a leading Berkeley, California, clinical ecologist and long-time consultant to the Environmental Illness Association.

The herbal tea being used is known by several common names, including *taheebo, lapacho,* and *ipe roxo.* Most of the commercial variety now comes from Brazil, but the authentic *lapacho* herb comes only from northeastern Argentina.

Brazil vs. Argentina: an herb war. While species of this tree (*Tabebuia impetiginosa* family Bignoniaceae) range from the jungles of Brazil to the grasslands of Patagonia, the best healing species, that with a purple flower, is found only in northeastern Argentina.

Only as a result of the war between Argentina and England was the shipment of this powerful herb interrupted. Brazilian foresters stepped in and began offering *their* species as the authentic *lapacho,* long reputed for healing properties since the time of the Incas.

Now it is true that the inner bark of the Brazilian trees is effective against candida, as testified by numerous clinicians in the United States. However, the Argentine lapacho is clearly more active medicinally.

Enter Agent Orange. In addition the Brazilian government is raping their tropical rain forests on an alarming scale, illegally using Agent Orange to defoliate trees and kill them, according to reports in the West German press. We fear that residues of this carcinogenic chemical are contaminating some shipments of Brazilian lapacho.

In contrast the Argentines have protected their coveted taheebo trees with a national "Save-A-Tree" program, enacted in 1953. In Argentina this medicinal bark is scraped from *living* trees only up to the height of a man, thereby allowing the trees to live. The Brazilian bark is scraped from dead trees, cut down for the lumber industry.

This is why we recommend that only Argentine lapacho be used as a medicinal tea.

Why does this bark work? The active chemical constituent found in the bark is called *lapachol*. It has shown strong activity against tumors* in tests with mice (*Cancer Chemotherapy Reports*, Part 2, Vol. 4 (4), December 1974) as well as antimalarial activity and the ability to kill the parasite *Schistosoma mansoni* (Austin 1974).

Interestingly, Chinese scientists have rediscovered an ancient folk remedy and are using it with great success in treating malaria. This "new" antimalarial drug, *Qinghaosu* (Artemisinin), "acts rapidly in restoring to consciousness comatose patients with cerebral malaria" (Klayman 1985). What is pertinent to our discussion of candidiasis is the fact that both this new antimalarial drug and the Argentine lapacho are botanically derived drugs in the space age. It is likely that nature produces chemicals that can destroy strains of micro-organisms resistant to synthetic drugs.

Chemically, lapachol is classified as a *quinone*, specifically a naphthoquinone. It is accepted knowledge that a drug's activity depends on how well and how rapidly it reaches the site of action within the body. Sometimes, though, derivatives of a drug, called *prodrugs*, can reach this site more rapidly and are then broken down to the active compound. In the case of lapachol, it was found that derivative compounds worked just this way. Lapachol itself was originally tested and found to be inactive in experimental tumor trials. Derivatives of lapachol, however, were found to

---

*Being active against tumors probably explains why this herb works in candidiasis. Both conditions are related to the immune system, in different pathways; but by stimulating immunity, the herb lessens the ability of the yeast to reproduce.

be very active in mouse leukemia and solid tumors, precisely those diseases that this tree bark is so famous for curing in South America (Koch 1961). It is likely that lapachol derivatives are formed when the bark is made into a hot water extract (tea) or when chemically converted into alcohol extracts (the "elixir" so popular in South American cancer clinics).

Dr. Norman Farnsworth of the University of Illinois confirms the value of this tree: "Taheebo undoubtedly contains a substance found to be highly effective against cancers. However, the substance was also found to be too toxic to be given to humans." As a result of the toxicity of this chemical extract, the National Cancer Institute ceased studies on this ancient Incan plant. But according to Dr. James Duke of the U.S. Department of Agriculture, the bark "is no more toxic than a lot of drugs now used to treat cancer in the U.S."*

Despite this reluctance on the part of the cancer establishment in the United States, extracts of taheebo are being used with great success in South America, especially against leukemia. I have reports of several leukemia cases in my files, including pre- and post-taheebo blood counts, and will provide them to the interested reader. A quick reference can be located in the 1975 *Journal of Medicinal Chemistry* (18:1159).

The powerful medicinal properties of this plant recommend its use as an over-the-counter remedy. Its utility in candidiasis has been attested to by hundreds of physicians in the United States and their approximately one million patients who are using the tea on a regular basis.

Why so many patients would elect to use this herbal remedy in an age of carefully synthesized drugs can be explained, perhaps, by the ineffectiveness of nystatin, the drug of "choice," against resistant strains of the offending fungal agent.

Taheebo, or Pau D'Arco, tea is generally available in the form of loose, air-dried bark, while a few companies offer it in the form of tea bags, tablets, and as a liquid extract.

Mathake: an antiyeast agent from Fiji. The Fiji Islands, located in the South Pacific and blessed with a near perfect climate, have a very diverse and unusual flora.

I had the good fortune of collecting medicinal plants in Fiji be-

*Both quotes are from the *Globe*, September 15, 1981.

tween 1969 and 1978 for the antitumor testing program of the U.S. National Cancer Institute. During these "plant hunts," I also learned of plants used by the local people for other ailments.* Many times I was given remedies for thrush, an almost commonplace yeast infection among island infants whose mothers no longer eat protective, traditional diets. *Mathake* means "thrush" in the Fijian language, and the tree with this name is the most frequently utilized remedy in Fiji for treating this uncomfortable yeast infection.

While extensive trials have not been conducted, clinical trials among patients of six physicians indicate that Mathake is far more effective than taheebo and requires much smaller quantities. As a point of reference, where one tablespoon of taheebo is needed to make one cup of tea for candidiasis, just a pinch of Mathake is necessary to make one very potent cup of tea.

At this time, the evidence for Mathake's usefulness is still folkloric and anecdotal. But because the "beastly yeast" is quite on the increase, Mathake's reputation in Fijian folk medicine is a strong recommendation for further analysis in the treatment of candidiasis.

If you are wondering whether *you* are affected by a candida overgrowth, you may want to have your physician order a laboratory analysis of your immune status (see Appendix 6). Appendix 4 lists yeast-containing foods that should be avoided if you are diagnosed with candidiasis and undertake a rotation diet to determine which of these foods may be particularly allergenic for you.

---

*Published as a book by the government press, Suva, as *Secrets of Fijian Medicine,* October 1984.

° 14 °

Immunity Against Allergies

IN AN IDEAL WORLD, people would not suffer from allergic reactions. In such a world, we would live where our people had lived for centuries and would be adapted to the flora, the food, and the other elements of the environment.

But human beings have shifted terrain, mixed their genes with strangers, and may no longer be adapted to many things in the environment.

Having traveled extensively in some remote Pacific islands where people have lived since at least A.D. 1200, where marriage outside the local population is extremely uncommon, and where traditional foods are still largely eaten, I am pleased to report that in such places the incidence of allergic disorders as we know them is practically nil.

But we, the peripatetic, who love exotic places and "interesting" foods, have our piper to pay. The piper is, all too often, paid in the currency of allergic symptoms.

ALLERGIC DISORDERS — COMMON AND UNCOMMON

Our environment is full of substances to which some of us are more sensitive than others. Treatment experts have only recently begun to accept the reality that allergies are much more widespread, and account for many more problems, than was once believed. In a world filled with not only "natural" allergens such as pollens, molds, insect venoms, and dust, but also new, manmade substances — such as synthetic fabrics, building materials, and food additives — it is no wonder that many people develop allergies.

Allergic symptoms are not limited to such obvious things as red eyes, runny nose, or rash. Allergy can produce symptoms that may go undetected deep within our bodies, or may become manifest in serious mental and emotional problems — a fact that is being increasingly recognized by people working with children who have behavioral disorders. Following are some of the more familiar forms that such hypersensitivities may take.

Hay fever (seasonal allergic rhinitis). If you are not a hay fever sufferer yourself, you probably know someone who suddenly comes down with itching nose and eyes, sneezing, and nasal stuffiness on otherwise "perfect" days. All these dramatic symptoms are produced by pollens in the air — pollens that are completely invisible and undetectable to the eye.

Hay fever is not well named, since it can be caused by any kind of pollen, not just hay; and while it has many symptoms, fever is not one of them. Seasonal allergic rhinitis is a more appropriate name, since the disease is an inflammatory reaction (rhinitis) of the nasal mucous membranes to the seasonal presence of one or more kinds of pollen.

Depending on what pollens a person is allergic to, hay fever symptoms will occur at different times of year. Tree pollens are generally present in the spring, grass pollens in early to midsummer, and weed pollens in late summer and early fall.

Hay fever is mediated by the immunoglobulin IgE. After repeated exposure to an allergen, the susceptible person becomes sensitized through a primary immune response in which the B cells and plasma cells produce IgE with allergen-specific IgE antibodies. Some of the IgE antibodies bind to receptor sites on mast cells in the submucosa of the nasal passages and sinuses. Subsequent exposure to the same allergen leads to the formation of an allergen/IgE complex on the mast cell surface, activating enzymes that release *chemical mediators* from the cell membrane and from granules discharged from the mast cell. Some of these mediators, such as histamine, act immediately, while others are slower acting. It is these mediators that produce the characteristic symptoms of the allergic reaction, through their action on the blood vessels, mucosa, and nerve endings. This typical "allergic reaction" is thought to be an attempt to rid the invading allergen from the body. Note that the reaction to an allergen is similar to the typical reaction to an invading antigen.

Nonseasonal allergic rhinitis. The same kinds of symptoms can be produced by allergens that are not seasonal in nature, but may be present at any time of year. House dust, mites, animal danders, or molds are among the allergens that can produce this type of atopic reaction.

Treatment of IgE-mediated allergic rhinitis, seasonal or non-seasonal, generally consists of three measures: avoidance of allergenic substances — which is sometimes very difficult; use of drugs, including antihistamines, decongestants, corticosteroids, and cromolyn; and immunotherapy, or desensitization shots. Since most drugs used to treat allergy have serious potential side effects, and since desensitization shots are expensive, inconvenient, and sometimes of questionable value, the unfortunate allergy-prone person is well advised to avoid exposure to allergens as much as possible, while building up healthy immune responsiveness through a nourishing diet and careful use of supplements. (See Chapters 5 and 6 for the specifics.)

Asthma. An estimated nine million Americans have asthma, and about two to three million of them are children. The disease is characterized by a persistent or intermittent blockage of the bronchioles, the multibranched air passageways that extend from the throat into the very small air sacs (alveoli) in the lungs where the exchange of oxygen and carbon dioxide takes place. The blockage of the airways can be caused by swelling of the bronchial mucous membranes, by tightening of the muscles that line the airways, and/or by mucus plugging the airways.

An asthmatic attack can be quite frightening, for victim and observer alike. The asthmatic may feel as if suffocating when trying to expel old air from the lungs. As the air flows through the narrowed tubes, it makes a characteristic whistling or wheezing sound. Sometimes an attack may consist mainly of dry coughing, with little or no wheezing. Asthmatic episodes may be mild or severe and may occur at any time, often at night. Eventually the episode subsides, from a few minutes to a few hours later.

While most asthma in children is allergic, only half of adult asthmatics have allergic problems. However, it is not unusual for adults to develop allergic asthma also.

Allergic asthma is also known as *extrinsic* asthma (meaning that it is caused by a response to an external allergen). Other triggers of asthma include lung infections, aspirin or other anti-inflammatory drugs, emotional stress, and violent exercise. *Exercise-induced asthma* is quite common, and in general the more strenuous the activity, the stronger is the asthmatic reaction. Swimming seems to be the most balanced kind of exercise, least likely to provide an attack in people with this problem.

Occupational asthma results from prolonged exposure to substances in the workplace, such as industrial fumes, dust, gases, animal dander (in the animal care and grooming professions), flour dust (especially wheat dust), carmine (a substance used in cosmetics), aluminum soldering flux (a hazard for electronics workers), formalin (a preservative used in the fur industry and in biological laboratories), and polyvinyl chloride fumes (encountered, for example, by meat wrappers), to name a few (Patterson 1980).

Eye allergies. Some allergic reactions produce specific symptoms in the eyes. In *contact dermatitis* and *dermato-conjunctivitis,* for example, the eyelids become thick and red, and the eyes burn and produce tears. The conjunctiva, or the transparent outer covering of the eyeball, is also affected in *acute allergic conjunctivitis,* an itching and swelling of the eyes in response to allergens in make-up. *Vernal conjunctivitis* ("spring" conjunctivitis) is a reaction to seasonal allergens, marked by an intense itching of the eyes, burning sensations, and/or sensitivity to light. *Uveitis* is an inflammation of the iris, the ciliary body, and the choroid portions of the inside of the eyeball (Patterson 1980).

Ear allergies. Various parts of the ear may also be affected by allergic reactions. The skin of the outer ear may develop contact dermatitis, an itching and flaking due to sensitivity to the metal in earrings, to hair sprays, or to other substances. The middle ear may become filled with fluid as a result of allergic reactions.

Insects can kill! For some highly susceptible people, an insect sting can be fatal, as a result of an *anaphylactic reaction* — a rapid allergic reaction in which several organ systems are affected simultaneously, sometimes bringing on death within minutes. Such deadly insect stings have been recognized for thousands of years.

A death from insect allergy is recorded in the tomb of the Egyptian king Menes, dating back to 2641 B.C.

To understand how insect stings can be fatal, we should look at the antigen-antibody reaction known as anaphylaxis. Anaphylaxis is a two-step process. First, a nontoxic antigen is introduced into the individual, through physical contact, injection, inhalation, ingestion, or an initial insect sting. This first dose is known as the *sensitizing dose*. This is followed by a latent period, during which antibodies are manufactured against that specific antigen. The second step occurs when the person is once again exposed to the antigen, in a *challenging or shocking dose* (as from a subsequent sting), which must be much stronger than the sensitizing dose. This shocking dose produces the anaphylactic response, which comes on within seconds or minutes of exposure. It may begin with a feeling of fright or a sense of impending doom, followed rapidly by symptoms in other organs. Common anaphylactic responses in humans include redness of the skin; bronchospasm and swelling of the larynx, making breathing difficult; nausea, vomiting, and diarrhea; chest pains and a drop in blood pressure. In severe cases, death may result through obstruction of breathing or vascular collapse. Anaphylactic shock may be an attempt to rid the body of the threatening antigen. For some reason an overreaction occurs.

The insects most commonly responsible for severe anaphylactic reactions are yellow jackets, honeybees, paper wasps, yellow hornets, boldfaced hornets, and fire ants. Other insects that have been known to provoke allergic reactions are mosquitoes, deer flies, horseflies, bedbugs, wheel bugs, kissing bugs, blister beetles, various caterpillars, fleas, lice, black widow spiders, brown recluse spiders, mites, ticks, and scorpions (Frazier 1969).

Since insects are everywhere in our environment, there is no way to avoid them. For the susceptible person, it could be very frightening to live in a world filled with stinging insects. People who are known to have severe anaphylactic reactions to insect stings may, therefore, carry with them epinephrine (adrenalin) and a syringe at all times. If they are stung by an insect, they administer an injection of epinephrine, which controls the anaphylactic reaction.

Other substances besides insect venom can also produce anaphylaxis. These include drugs — such as protein products, certain antibiotics, anesthetics, and salicylates — and foods, including legumes, nuts, berries, seafoods, and egg albumin.

Food allergies. It has been known for a long time that food allergies can produce gastrointestinal distress and skin rashes. More recently it has been recognized that food allergies can also produce a whole range of symptoms in virtually every part of the body — including the nervous system. When the brain is involved in an allergic reaction, serious emotional and mental symptoms can result. Table 16 lists the chronological order in which various food allergy symptoms may appear.

Children may develop allergies to many kinds of foods. The most common are cow's milk, hen's eggs, fish, red meat, poultry, cereals, nuts, legumes, fruits, cabbage, cauliflower, tomato, potato, onion, chocolate, shellfish, and additives (Soothill 1983). Adults may be allergic to the same foods, as well as pork and bacon, cheese, yeast, tea, and coffee (Lessof 1983). (Table 5 in Chapter 5 provides a detailed list of common food allergens.)

Food additives are increasingly being recognized as a source of allergic reactions. With more than three thousand synthetic and natural substances used as additives in processed foods, susceptible people must read labels carefully. Used to preserve foods, improve their appearance or taste, common food additives include acids, bases, bleaches, buffers, colors, dyes, preservatives, emulsifiers, stabilizers, flavorings, solvents, phosphates, and many others (Eagle 1981).

Certain naturally occurring amines in foods can also cause problems for sensitive people, producing a rise in blood pressure and other symptoms. Common offenders are histamine and tyramine. Tyramine, formed as a result of fermentation or of microbial action during aging, is found in certain cheeses; fermented drinks such as wine, beer, and ale; salted dried fish, pickled herring, meat extracts, and stored liver (Weiner 1981). Histamine-rich foods include sauerkraut; dried pork; wine, beer, and other fermented drinks; stored fish; sausage; tomato; and spinach (Moneret-Vantrin 1983). These blood-vessel dilators (amines) can be particularly dangerous for people who are taking MAO-inhibitor drugs, such as certain medications for treating depression. Even small amounts of amine-rich foods can produce serious rises

TABLE 16

Order of Appearance of Food Allergy Symptoms

Symptom(s)	Elapsed Time (after ingesting offending food)
Heartburn and indigestion	within ½ hour
Headache	within 1 hour
Rhinitis and asthma	within 1 hour
Bloating of stomach and diarrhea	3–4 hours
Hives and rashes	6–12 hours
Noticeable weight gain from fluid retention	12–15 hours
Fits, confusion, and other mental aberrations	12–24 hours
Mouth ulcers; aching joints, muscles, or back	48–96 hours

Source: Eagle, 1981

in blood pressure in people using these drugs. Histamines in foods also commonly produce headaches in susceptible people (Weiner 1981).

The obvious way to avoid an allergic reaction to a food is to refrain from eating it. Many people have food allergies of which they are not aware. Food allergens can be identified through various forms of testing, including skin testing, sublingual testing (placing a tiny amount of the suspect substance under the tongue), and rotation diets, which eliminate suspect foods and then reintroduce them one by one. A recently developed diagnostic tool is cytotoxic testing, which observes the interaction between a suspect substance and a sample of the person's blood cells.

Drug allergies. People have adverse reactions to medications for many different reasons, one of which is allergy. Some two hundred thousand patients in hospitals suffer allergic reactions to their medication each year, while another fifty thousand are hospitalized to treat allergic drug reactions developed outside the hospital. In addition there may be more than one million drug allergy reactions that occur away from the hospital each year.

Drug allergies can produce many different symptoms, depending on the drug, the dosage, and the person's sensitivity. Some common drug allergy reactions include: anaphylaxis, fever, skin

250 · DISEASE AND IMMUNITY

eruptions, bronchial asthma, blood changes, digestive disturbances, liver and kidney problems, inflammation of blood vessels
and connective tissue, and neurological problems (De Swarte
1980).

Penicillin is a very common cause of allergic reaction. It can
produce virtually every kind of allergic symptom known, with the
most frequent being a skin rash. Approximately one out of every
ten thousand courses of penicillin treatment results in anaphylaxis, which accounts for about three hundred deaths each year in
the United States. As with other anaphylactic reactions, that produced by penicillin brings on immediate symptoms; rashes or
other symptoms that appear days or weeks later are not as serious,
and the symptoms will subside if the drug is discontinued. It is
because of penicillin's ability to produce severe allergic reactions
that your doctor always asks if you are allergic to it when you are
being treated with antibiotics.

Other drugs frequently linked with allergic reactions include
aspirin, sulfa drugs, antituberculous drugs, antimalarials, seda-
tive-hypnotics, anticonvulsants, anesthetics, phenolphthalein, antipsychotic tranquilizers, antihypertensive agents, antiarrhythmic
agents, antisera and vaccines, organ extracts (such as insulin),
heavy metals (gold), antithyroid drugs, barbiturates, and hormones (De Swarte 1980). If you are placed on a medication, you
should be alert for any unusual symptoms that may appear. They
may be signs of an allergic reaction, and you may need to discontinue the medication and find another to which you are not sensitive.

Another important method of countering drug side effects is to
know which nutrients are depleted by various drugs and to take
these nutrients as supplements. For example, prednisone (a synthetic corticosteroid) depletes body stores of vitamins B_{12} and C,
as well as inducing zinc and potassium deficiency. This can lead
to tingling in the limbs, even a loss of feeling. To avoid these side
effects, the affected nutrients must be supplemented when the
drug is taken.*

*The chart "Fifty Common Prescription Drugs and the Nutrients They Af-
fect" can be found in a previous book and will not be reproduced here; see
Weiner and Goss, *Nutrition Against Aging* (1983).

ALLERGY TESTING

Medical allergists use skin tests to determine which allergens are causing a person problems. The test consists of introducing a small sample of purified allergen under the skin of the subject. Usually, many different allergens are applied at the same time, at different locations on the skin. A positive reaction — consisting of localized redness, swelling, and/or itching at the point where the allergen was introduced — indicates that the subject is allergic to that particular allergen.

Clinical ecologists use sublingual testing, in which a minute amount of a suspect substance is placed under the person's tongue. A positive reaction may occur very rapidly and may include pronounced emotional and behavioral symptoms.

Allergy testing is important for several reasons. It is relatively easy to avoid some allergens, and so if the guilty substance turns out to be, for example, poison ivy, then the individual can simply make sure not to come into contact with it. However, it may be something that is virtually unavoidable, such as ragweed pollen. In such cases, the sufferer can be immunized against the pollen by a series of injections.

IMMUNIZATION AGAINST ALLERGIES

Hyposensitization, or immunization, consists of a series of injections of the offending allergens. Several allergens may be mixed together into a single injection per treatment. The initial injection is small, with succeeding ones growing larger and less frequent. The object is for the immune system to become tolerant of the allergen, so that the levels of allergen that formerly prompted an allergic reaction are no longer harmful. Such a series of injections may stretch over a period of months or years, depending upon the individual's particular situation.

This kind of immunotherapy is effective in reducing the symptoms of hay fever (seasonal pollen allergy) and also appears to help in cases of mold and dust allergy. It is less effective in other allergic situations.

TREATING ALLERGIES THROUGH CLINICAL ECOLOGY

You should be well aware by now of this book's repeated emphasis on the use of the three elements of immune stimulation for a wide variety of problems. Fortunately, confirmation that at least one of these elements, nutrition, works to help the allergy sufferer comes to us from reliable sources.

The first rule of "clinical ecology," coined by Theron Randolph, M.D.,* is to *eliminate* the offending food, chemical, or other source of allergic reaction. This may not be accomplished easily. Some people are so sickened by chemical toxins, which may appear in every aspect of their life (homes, cars, airplanes, etc.), that they must be treated at special ecology units. For example, Brookhaven Medical Center, in Dallas, Texas — directed by William Rea, M.D., an eminent cardiovascular surgeon and allergist — specializes in creating an allergen-free environment. In such an environment, devoid of all known and suspected allergens (from house dust to soap, fumes, odors, and specially prepared foods), the patient is gradually exposed to single suspected foods and chemicals, one at a time. After it is determined which items are inciting the reactions, the patient is sent home and instructed in a new reality of abstinence and withdrawal.

In addition to abstaining from possible allergens, or moving away from areas that cause allergic reactions, some people have learned that various nutrients stimulate their resistance to allergens and can effectively stop or retard an attack.

Multiple food and chemical allergies are common to patients with deficient immune systems. When allergies become severe, the sufferer experiences a breakdown in immune recognition and may constantly react to foreign proteins found in the air, food, water, and even their own body!

While avoidance of all potential contaminants is often recommended by clinical ecologists to people with such deficient immune systems, few patients can afford to relocate to the ocean or

---

*Dr. Randolph was the pioneer who created the field of clinical ecology. A board-certified allergist, he broke with conventional allergists in recognizing the extent of environmentally induced allergies.

to an environment where the air is relatively pure. While not fatal, such "ecological" illness is often a disease they must learn to live with.

Fortunately, as we have discussed throughout this book, there are a number of nutritional factors that enhance immune function. These can provide relief for patients with multiple food and chemical allergies. A Berkeley, California, group that makes nutrients for people with allergies has specialized in "clean" vitamins and minerals.* Two of their products, appropriately named *T Cell Formula* and *B Cell Formula,* contain immune-enhancing nutrients. The T cell product is derived from lambs, while the B cell one is derived from extracts of animal spleen and bone marrow. Thymosin and other hormones in B Cell Formula can not be synthesized and must be derived from the thymus gland of young animals. The reason this formula is classified as a food is that papaya enzyme is used to liberate the fat-soluble hormone, unlike drugs of this nature which are chemically created.

Several physicians using thymosin have found that this natural substance increases the number of T cells in patients with deficient immune systems and that it can partially restore immune competence. In addition an improvement of the helper to suppressor ratio of T cells was also observed in some cases (Robert Da Prato, M.D., pers. com. 1985).

---

*This group, Arteria, Inc., can be contacted at P.O. Box 5277, Berkeley, CA 94705.

PART IV

ACHIEVING FREEDOM FROM CARE

Overview

"Immunity" can mean "freedom from obligation." In the sense of this book, the concept means that once you do what you can to incorporate the recent findings about stimulating your immune system into your way of life, you should no longer worry about illness. That is the true meaning of immunity and the purpose of this book — to free you from inordinate care about disease.

In the beginning, we stated that "the word itself is magic." If you look at the principal elements that, when incorporated into your life, become a *unified* immunity program, the "magic" becomes science.

The next chapter brings us to the means for incorporating these elements into your life and concludes with a conceptual leap that just might help you achieve a powerful control over your health and vigor.

15

Unifying Mind, Body, and Motion

BEING THE INTERNAL DEFENSE system of the body, your immune system obviously guards against foreign invaders. When a foreign organism or substance breaks through the first line of defenses, through mechanisms already explained the immune system begins to neutralize, destroy, or isolate the threatening elements.

We have seen how this works. The thymus, bone marrow, spleen, and lymph all act in harmony to defend the body. Going *beyond* defensive procedures, we can begin to see that the immune system also produces substances that act like drugs to create the healing that follows illness. Endorphins, acting like opiates to calm us, are produced through subtle mind/body interactions. Adrenalin, thyroxin, testosterone, estrogens, and hundreds of other hormones secreted by the endocrine glands should be seen as related, if not interconnected, to the immune system.

What we call "the immune system" has been isolated here from other components of the human miracle in order to define the components of immunity and describe what they do. But we have to remember that the whole organism works as one vast unit. This is the meaning of the word "holistic" (which now seems so out of date). Yes, we can define separate anatomical and physiological entities as elements belonging to the immune system. And we can also see how interconnected are these cellular products of defense with the cellular substances produced by other systems, all utilized by the body for living and healing. Endocrine glands produce hormones, and these are strongly related to mind and body activities and controls. But even our "lowly" saliva is a critical component of digestion, without which the digestion of starches would be difficult, if not impossible. This would in turn cause other systems to compensate with yet other substances, and so on. The point is, while we can separate one system from another for purposes of learning how they operate and how to maximize their operational capacity, the borderline between purely defensive substances and purely offensive ones is quite imaginary. Both types of substances are engaged in critical operations at all times.

In this broader context, the immune system can be seen as an internal apothecary. Utilizing this analogy, we can see that the elements described throughout the book are means for deciding which life-saving "drugs" to stock, how to keep the "shelves" of our apothecary shop filled, and how to move the drugs to those places that most need them.

STRATEGIES FOR MAXIMUM IMMUNITY

Look again at the building blocks in Chapter 1. The Master Sheet is a condensation of new findings in using mind to control our state of health. Whichever one of many different "mind" techniques (biofeedback, meditation, prayer, etc.) you utilize, you will find that the nine inner cubes of this building block concisely define the kinds of beneficial results you can expect to achieve. If you have "not had a major illness in years," have "never suffered from allergies," and you do "not feel like an 'outsider' " — and also rate highly in the other cubes of the Master Sheet — more than likely you are in control of your own psychic powers as they affect your state of health. By working on gaining more insight, more control, over your mind, you will score even higher in the months and years ahead.

The Drugs, Sex, and Intimacy building block is closely related to the Master Sheet because it is also associated with control over emotions. But, as you have seen throughout this book, the emotions are intimately tied to your nutritional state as well as your degree of physical activity. In the case of this block, we look at how much reliance you place on titrating yourself to a level of calm by using drugs, alcohol, tobacco, and sensual interludes.

Insert your new scores from the building blocks in Chapter 1 and compute your total score. Then check the rating scale that follows.

```
                    ┌──────────────────────┐
                    │ Mind/Body            │
                    │ Connections          │
                    │                      │
                    │                      │
                    │ Your score _____  │
        ┌───────────┴──────────┬───────────┴──────────┐
        │ Drugs, Sex, and Inti-│ Avoiding Unhealthy   │
        │ macy Component       │ Food Component       │
        │                      │                      │
        │                      │                      │
        │ Your score _____  │ Your score _____  │
┌───────┴──────────┬───────────┴──────────┬───────────┴──────────┐
│ Healthful Food Com-│ Exercise Component  │ The Vitamin and Min- │
│ ponent            │                     │ eral Component       │
│                   │                     │                      │
│                   │                     │                      │
│ Your score _____ │ Your score _____   │ Your score _____    │
└───────────────────┴─────────────────────┴──────────────────────┘
```

Your total score _____

RATING YOUR IM.Q.

Scores between 230–256 = A+; 190–229 = A; 170–189 = B+; 150–169 = B; 140–149 = B–; 130–139 = Average; 120–129 = D; below 119 = F.

Although this is only a rough gauge of your immunity, it should begin to help you see the kinds of things that go into building a healthy immune system. For a medically accurate reading of your immune status, we suggest you see a physician, who can order the appropriate tests.

What you are probably searching for (if you do overrely on these substitutes) is a shared intimacy. This "intimacy," by the way, does not have to be experienced with another adult in the sense of marriage. It can be with a grandparent, a child, a neighbor. The key element is *feeling* that you are close to that person, needed by that person, and able to receive from them. This block, like the others, is a subjective guide to self. Through time, through thought, you can learn to throw away your "crutches" and find the true meaning of a meaningful life: another person, or other people.

The Avoiding Unhealthy Food Component, the Healthful Food Component, and the Exercise Component are straightforward building blocks with inner cubes that need not be discussed. The Vitamin and Mineral Component offers a convenient guide to a model supplement program. But please also refer to the nutrition chapters, where you will find suggestions for establishing *your* individual needs for extra vitamins and minerals. You may, after proper analysis, discover that you need more of certain nutrients and less of others.

Looking back, we can see that your Im.Q., or Immunity Quotient, can be calculated by adding together all the scores from the building blocks on the previous page. The total scores have been equated to a simple scheme. Admittedly, this is a highly subjective means for approximating your relative state of immune readiness. But, taken together with a laboratory analysis (see Appendix 6), it becomes a tool for use in gaining and maintaining immunity.

GETTING THE MOST FROM FOODS

The last point that needs to be mentioned concerns the question of extracting the most from the foods we eat. We begin with the concept of "food fascism," which seems to be the order of the day.

OVERCOMING FOOD FASCISM

Feed all things with food convenient for them. . . . The food of thy soul is light and space; feed it then on light and space. But the food of the body is champagne and oysters; feed it then on champagne and oysters.

Herman Melville

Not for everyone, Melville's champagne and oyster diet is a useful reminder that one man's meat may be another's poison. Food fascism is what we call those all too popular tractates of dietary "dos" and "don'ts." It is simply bad science to prescribe and proscribe diets for whole populations of readers. Ethnic differences alone would render such dietary absolutes useless if not harmful. Consider also that *individual* differences even within homogeneous ethnic groups explain why some people love meat and others do not, or some are nauseated by goat cheese, others not, and so on, down to the simple glass of milk, which is now a matter of some controversy.

It simply is not advisable to attempt to have millions of people conform to a set of rigid dietary guidelines that may not suit them — ethnically, aesthetically, or idiosyncratically.

SOURCES OF MICRONUTRIENTS:
SUPPLEMENTS OR FOOD?

Now the question arises: how are we going to get all the vitamins and minerals we need? Can we get them from our food alone, or do we need to take vitamin supplements? Although the first source of adequate nutrition must be our diet, we must recognize that our food supply is not what it used to be. Moreover, because we have switched from a more active to a more sedentary lifestyle in the twentieth century, we do not need to consume the same number of calories that people did in the past. This is one reason obesity has become a major problem in modern civilization.

Although we may need to cut back on our caloric intake, our micronutrient requirements may remain the same. It stands to reason, then, that we need to rely on some supplementation in order to obtain the vital minerals and vitamins that would otherwise be carried by calorie-laden foods.

In evaluating your supplement needs, remember that the RDAs, or Recommended Dietary Allowances, for a given nutrient do *not* reflect the needs of any given individual. Your own individual requirements for these nutrients may be much higher, depending on your overall nutritional status, your state of health, and other factors. Use how you feel, your relative stress level, and other *subjective* gauges as your first guide to nutrient supplementation. Then, for specifics, you may want to have your doctor order hair and serum analyses of your vitamin and mineral levels.

NUTRIENTS IN VEGETARIAN FOODS

Much of the emphasis in this book has been on increasing the amount of fruits, vegetables, grains, and other nutrient-dense foods, while decreasing the amount of flesh foods. But learning which vegetable foods to select in order to assure yourself adequate amounts of critical nutrients such as calcium, zinc, folic acid, and vitamin B$_{12}$ requires knowing specific nutrients found in vegetarian foods.

Most tables presently available do not include foods that vegetarians commonly eat. Have you ever tried to find the amount of calcium in black beans, the iron content of mung beans, the zinc in garbanzo beans, or the potassium in bamboo shoots?

Consider the nutrient value of tofu. Tofu, or bean curd, is a wonderful source of complete protein: while low in sodium and low in fat, it is quite a good source of complex carbohydrates and magnesium. For the purposes of this book, it can be considered a wonder food and can be added to your diet as you cut down on meats and sugars. The Japanese and Chinese have used this food since antiquity. Made from soybean curds that are pressed from soaked ground soybeans, tofu can be prepared in many creative ways, with a variety of flavors and textures.

Using the nutrients table for vegetarian foods in Appendix 7, found in the back of this book, you can now, for the first time, determine how much of the critical nutrients you are getting from bamboo shoots, various beans, esoteric cheeses, whole-meal flours, goat's milk, yogurt, water chestnuts, and a host of other nutrient-dense foods. Appendix 7 should help you plan your meals with new confidence.

BALANCING AMINO ACIDS

Amino acids are the subunits of proteins. When you eat a source of protein (meat, eggs, legumes, etc.), your body breaks the protein down into its constituent amino acids through the action of enzymes (which are also proteins). There are about twenty amino acids that the human body requires; of these, there are eight that our bodies are unable to manufacture themselves.

These eight are referred to as the "essential" amino acids. A deficiency in any essential amino acid affects the immune system by depressing specific immune functions, as has been demonstrated in numerous studies (Beisel et al. 1981).

Since protein is the material used to build and repair body cells, it is very important for you to take in complete protein, containing all eight essential amino acids. Animal products such as fish, meat, poultry, eggs, and dairy products all contain complete protein, while most vegetable sources supply incomplete protein. Soybeans are an exception, supplying all eight essential amino acids, and so soy products are a reasonable source of dietary protein for most people.

It is possible, through paying careful attention to the amino acid content of various vegetable products, to obtain all essential amino acids from vegetable sources. For example, whole-grain rice combined with beans supplies all essential amino acids. In many ethnic diets from around the world, such combinations of grains and legumes have become the staple sources of all necessary protein in the diet.

Thus, through well-thought-out and carefully conceived food combinations, it is quite possible to receive excellent nutrition on a strictly vegetarian diet. In fact, such a diet may actually be superior for many people. One researcher has observed: "An inescapable fact is that vegetarians are not only just as healthy as others, but in some important ways healthier, with a substantially lower incidence of heart attacks, strokes, intestinal disorders and some forms of cancer" (Turner 1982).

You do not need to be a nutrition expert in order to obtain all the essential amino acids in your diet, even if you are not eating meat, fish, or poultry. As long as you are consuming dairy products or eggs, you are assured of receiving all eight essential amino acids. This so-called lacto-ovo-vegetarian diet is especially recommended for small children, as opposed to a strict vegetarian diet.

MEAT, POULTRY, AND FISH

Because of the principle of biological magnification, discussed in Chapter 5, it is wise to cut down on your consumption of *all* animal protein. This does not mean that you should entirely avoid meat and seafood; rather, cut back on red meat and substitute *moderate* amounts of poultry and fish. It is very important to avoid the processed meats such as frankfurters, bologna, salami, ham, bacon, and others that are preserved with nitrites; this chemical is a potent anti-immunity compound.

FOOD PREPARATION

Many cooking methods that we use today can place us at risk for disease. When fish or meat is smoked or broiled, for example, carcinogens can be produced. Frying in fat, and particularly deep frying, also produces harmful cancer-causing substances, especially when the same oil is reheated repeatedly. Charcoal-broiled steaks, although they may taste delicious, also contain powerful mutagens produced by the charcoal-broiling process. For maximum protection of your immune functioning, all these cooking methods should be avoided.

While red meats are generally discouraged, proper preparation can reduce their risk factors. Proper preparation means choosing meats with less fat, trimming off all visible fat, and cooking for longer periods of time (to remove more fat). Poultry is preferable to red meats due to its lower fat and cholesterol content, and fish is superior to poultry for the same reasons (Germann 1977), while also carrying protective nutrients. Remember, those Alaskan Eskimos who still subsist on salmon have almost *no* heart disease.

Unfortunately, you generally can not just look up the vitamin and mineral content of your foods on a chart to see if your diet is providing adequate amounts of these important nutrients. Whether you are actually *absorbing* these nutrients in your body will depend on a number of factors, including for example, whether you are taking any medications that might interfere with the absorption of certain micronutrients.

Cooking and processing methods also have a great influence on the micronutrients in your foods. Fruits and vegetables should be bought fresh whenever possible, and generally the best way to eat them is raw. If you must use packaged vegetables, use frozen rather than canned; modern freezing methods preserve most of the nutrient value of the fresh food, while the heat used in canning destroys important vitamins.

Vegetables should be cooked with the skins left on to save nutrients, and the skins should be eaten whenever possible. Steaming is the cooking method of choice, while quick stir frying in a very small amount of oil will also retain most of the nutrients. Boiling not only destroys vitamins through heat, but also removes the nutrients from the vegetables, bringing them into the cooking water, which should be saved and used for gravies, soups, and stocks.

FINAL NOTES

That nature heals can not be questioned. That she heals best when augmented by sound stimuli is the thrust of this book. We are not passive animals when it comes to illness and healing. Yes, some of our synthetic drugs *are* truly lifesaving, and they must be seen as *part* of the overall healing picture. The immune-enhancing nutrients, and other components described for maximizing immunity, are best when incorporated as *preventive* measures — before illness appears. Should you feel yourself weakening because of stress or exposure, these immune stimulants should be looked at as a first line of defense. Should you fall ill and require the care of a physician and the attendant drugs, the tips for stimulating immunity outlined here should be maintained, as part of an overall program of recovery.

For a decade now, things "natural" have been scorned, relegated to the past, as something antiquated in an age of high technology. What was once the vanguard, in the 1960s, natural healing products such as nutrients and herbs, were somehow suddenly passé. And now we find ourselves in the midst of a growing revival of interest in things natural. With the publication in *Science* magazine, moreover on the front cover, of a major new treatment for malaria derived from an ancient Chinese folk remedy, the world of science began again to look to nature for her healing secrets (see *Science,* May 31, 1985). The microbe that brought about the wrenching fevers of malaria had become resistant to the "wonder" drugs produced by our best laboratories. Chinese scientists decided to resist the romance with biotechnology and genetically engineered drugs. Instead they took a common herb, a relative of wormwood (*Artemisia annua*), long recommended by their ancient healers, isolated from the leaves of the plant a substance, and found it a highly effective treatment for fever and malaria. This discovery, more than any other single factor, revitalized the interest in natural products.

The point of this anecdote is to emphasize the powers of nature and make the link to our own natural healers within. Instead of looking *outside* of our bodies for healing properties, we should conceptualize the pharmacy within and clearly see that by providing the shelves with the necessary starter compounds in the form of required nutrients, we can use our mind to make the inner drugs.

That is the story of natural healing.

APPENDICES

LIMITED
GLOSSARY

REFERENCES

INDEX

Appendix 1

T Cell Ratios in Some Disorders

	Helper to Suppressor Ratio
Normal	1.8 : 1 (approx.)
Disease	
Cold hemagglutinin disease	2.05 : 1
Warm antibody disease	
• without steroids	3.28 : 1
• with steroids	1.94 : 1
Systemic lupus erythematosus	1.51 : 1
Myasthenia gravis	
• before thymectomy	2.41 : 1
• after thymectomy	3.82 : 1
Membranous glomerulonephritis	2.50 : 1
Buerger's disease	2.33 : 1
Chronic active hepatitis	
• HBs + (Hepatitis B antibodies present)	1.34 : 1
• HBs − (Hepatitis B antibodies *not* present)	2.21 : 1
Multiple sclerosis	
• remission	1.77 : 1
• acute phases	2.50 : 1
• progressive form	2.81 : 1
Leprosy	
• without erythema nodosum leprosum	1.64 : 1
• with erythema nodosum leprosum	2.91 : 1
• tuberculoid form	1.86 : 1
Cutaneous lymphoma	
• Sézary syndrome	greater than 4.0 : 1
• mycosis fungoides	3.80 : 1
AIDS	(approx.) 1 : 1 (or less)

Source: Bach and Bach, 1981

Appendix 2

Nutrients You Can Take to Influence
Your Nervous System

Nutrient Precursor	Abundance/ Source	Neurotransmitter	Related Effects
Tryptophan (amino acid)	1% of all dietary proteins	Serotonin	In normal people: • Decreases alertness • Hastens sleep onset • Decreases appetite (especially for carbohydrates) • Diminishes pain sensitivity In disease states: • Assists in treating depression, obesity, insomnia
Tyrosine (amino acid)	5% of all dietary proteins	Catecholamines • norepinephrine • epinephrine • dopamine	In normal people: • Reduces stress • Increases subjective vigor in aged In disease states: • Normalizes blood pressure • Reduces symptoms in early Parkinson's disease • Assists in treating depression
Choline	Component of lecithin (phosphatidylcholine) found in egg yolks, soy products, and liver	Acetylcholine	In disease states: • Under experimental evaluation in tardive dyskinesia, long-term treatment of Alzheimer's disease, mania, ataxias

Source: Weisburd, 1984

Appendix 3

Fats and Immunity

Immune function	High fat intake and/or obesity	Polyunsaturated fatty acid deficit	Polyunsaturated fatty acid excess	Cholesterol excess
Host susceptibility to infection	Increased			Increased
Lymphoid tissues	Relative decrease in size		Thymic and splenic weight loss	
In vitro T and B cell responses	Altered surface membrane fluidity		Suppressed response to mitogens; altered killer cell activity	Diminished cytotoxic activity; diminished response to mitogens
Serum immunoglobulin concentrations		Some may increase		
Antibody production		Impaired		Variable; may be suppressed
Splenic plaque cells		Diminished production		
Graft survival		Shortened	Prolonged	
Delayed dermal hypersensitivity				Suppressed
Susceptibility to induced allergic encephalitis		Increased susceptibility	Decreased susceptibility	
Neutrophil chemotaxis	May be slowed			
Neutrophil phagocytic activity	May be depressed			
Neutrophil bactericidal activity	May be depressed			
Macrophages		May alter motility		Foam cell appearance
Reticuloendothelial system	Clearance slowed		Clearance accelerated	Effects inconsistent
Other				Oxidized metabolites may be immunosuppressive

Source: Beisel, 1982

Appendix 4
Foods Containing Yeast

This list is intended for use as part of a rotation diet to determine which of these foods may be particularly allergenic for you. As with all such lists, this one is partial. Carefully look at all labels and check the contents of canned and packaged foods.

Enriched flour
(with vitamins from yeast)
Breads
Crackers
Pastries
Pretzels
Rolls
Cookies
Cake and cake mix
Pita pockets
Cracker crumbs
Flat breads
Rye crisps (some)

Malted cereals
Doughnuts
Oatmeal
Barley cereal

Cheese
Buttermilk
Cottage cheese
Yogurt
Fermented milk

Mushrooms
Truffles
Chili peppers
Pickled vegetables
Olives
Sauerkraut
Horseradish
Pickles

Ketchup
Mayonnaise
Salad dressing
Barbecue sauce
Tomato sauce

Mince pies
Malted candies

Condiments
Vinegars:
    Apple cider
    Distilled
    Grape
    Gin
    Pear
    Wine
Cooking wines and sherries

Fortified milk (with
    vitamins from yeast)
Beer
Brandy
Wine
Whiskey
Rum
Vodka
Root beer
Malted milk drinks
Citrus fruit juices
(frozen or canned)

All vitamins with ingredients
    derived from yeast
Protein powder supplements
Yeast powder or flakes

Appendix 5

Viral Cancers in Animals

Virus	Natural Host	Cancer Association*
Bovine papilloma virus	Bovine	Carcinoma
Shope papilloma virus	Rabbit	Carcinoma
Polyomavirus	Mouse	Adenocarcinoma in multiple tissues
SV40	Monkey	Fibrosarcoma, glioma, leukemia, lymphoma, osteosarcoma, and reticulum cell sarcoma (hamster)
Adenoviruses (human)	Human	Transformation and oncogenesis (fibrosarcoma) demonstrated for many adenoviruses in several species of target cells and/or hosts, respectively
Herpesvirus saimiri	Squirrel monkey	Leukemia, lymphoma (marmoset)
H. ateles	Spider monkey	(T-lymphocytic)
H. papio	Baboon	Lymphoproliferative (marmoset)
Guinea pig herpes-virus	Guinea pig	Leukemia, transformation
H. sylvilagus	Cottontail rabbit	Lymphoproliferative, lymphoma
Marek's disease virus	Chicken	Lymphoma
Lucké's herpesvirus	Leopard frog	Renal adenocarcinoma
Yaba monkey virus	Rhesus monkey	Superficial tumors of limbs
Shope fibroma virus	Cottontail rabbit	Fibroma (benign, noninvasive)
Myxomatosis virus	Rabbit	Fibroma (benign, invasive)
Rous sarcoma virus	Chicken	Sarcoma
Avian leukemia virus	Chicken	Leukemia
Others (100)	Multiple species	Variety of tumors
Woodchuck hepatitis	Woodchuck	Hepatocellular carcinoma

*Animal or site or type of associated cancer is contained in parentheses.

Source: Lynch, Schuelke, and O'Hara, 1984

Appendix 6

LABORATORY TESTS FOR IMMUNE STATUS

It is now possible, using highly sophisticated laboratory techniques, to assess the condition of your immune system. At the same time, these techniques have resulted in the development of characteristic immunological profiles or "fingerprints" of many immune disorders, aiding in the recognition and treatment of these problems. Such laboratory tests evaluate either for the cellular (T and B cell) or the immunoglobulin composition of the blood.

The cellular evaluation is known as *cellular immune assay*. It measures the percentage of T cells, B cells, T helper cells, T suppressor cells, and null cells (these may be T cell precursors); the total count of T cells, B cells, and null cells; and the helper to suppressor ratio. By measuring these white cell subsets, the tests are able to determine numerical abnormalities in the various types of cells and in the helper to suppressor ratio, which may be related to functional abnormalities.

The second type of testing looks for autoantibodies and is used to detect a breakdown in the regulatory arm of the immune system, which may indicate autoimmune disease. The particular autoantibodies sought — those that would indicate autoimmune disease — are called antinuclear, mitochondrial, parietal cell, basement membrane, reticulin, brush border, smooth muscle, canalicular, and glomerular basement membrane antibodies. Each of these autoantibodies attacks a specific body component. In the order already named, their respective autoantigens are the nuclei (home of the cellular genetic material) of target cells (a kind of red cell); the mitochondria (cellular "powerhouses" where sugar is converted to energy during respiration) of target cells; the cells of the parietal lobe of the brain; the deep layer of the skin; other connective tissue; the microvilli (microscopic outfoldings of the intestinal linings that absorb nutrients); the bone cell connections; and kidney cells.

Your physician can also send samples of your blood to specialized laboratories that may detect the presence of many other ailments, such as cancer, diabetes, heart disease, respiratory disease, tissue disease, gastrointestinal disease, and genitourinary disease. The results of such autoantibody testing are combined with the cellular immune assay results for a total picture of your health, including predisease states. If you are in the early stages of any of the diseases tested for, these assays will detect the signs.

Source: Immunodiagnostic Laboratories, 400 29th Street, Suite 508, Oakland, CA 94609 kindly provided the above summary.

Appendix 7

Nutrients in Vegetarian Foods (per 100 grams edible)

food	water	energy	pro- tein	fat	carbo- hydrate	cal- cium	phos- phorus	iron
	%	kcal	←		gm	→	←		mg
acerola juice								
raw	94.3	21	0.4	0.3	4.8	10	9	0.5
alfalfa sprouts								
raw	91.14	29	3.99	0.69	3.78	32	70	0.96
amaranth								
cooked	91.49	21	2.11	0.18	4.11	209	72	2.26
bamboo shoots								
raw	91.	27	2.6	0.3	5.2	13	59	0.5
beans and peas								
cowpeas — black-eyed	71.8	109	8.1	0.8	18.15	28	119	1.43
broad beans	83.7	56	4.8	0.5	10.1	18	73	1.5
peas — edible pod	89.91	42	3.27	0.23	7.05	42	55	1.97
lima beans	67.17	123	6.81	0.32	23.64	32	130	2.45
pinto beans	58.01	162	9.31	0.48	30.88	52	—	2.71
soybeans	68.6	141	12.35	6.4	11.05	145	158	2.5
broccoli	90.2	29	2.97	0.28	5.57	114	48	1.15
cabbage								
raw	92.52	24	1.21	0.18	5.37	47	246	0.56
carrots								
cooked	87.38	45	1.09	0.18	10.48	31	30	0.62
cheese								
brick	41.11	371	23.24	29.68	2.79	674	451	.43
Camembert	51.8	300	19.8	24.26	.46	388	347	.33
Edam	41.56	357	24.99	27.8	1.43	731	536	.44
feta	55.22	264	14.21	21.28	4.09	492	337	.65
Gouda	41.46	356	24.94	27.44	2.22	700	546	.24
Gruyère	33.19	413	29.81	32.34	.36	1011	605	—
Limburger	48.42	327	20.05	27.25	.49	497	393	.13

potas-sium	zinc	vit. A	thiamin	ribo-flavin	niacin	vit. C	folacin
→		RE	←		mg	→	mcg
97	—	51	0.02	0.06	0.4	1600	—
79	0.92	16	0.076	0.126	0.481	8.2	36
641	—	277	0.02	0.134	0.559	41.1	—
533	—	2	0.15	0.07	0.6	4	—
420	0.79	64	0.068	0.107	1.073	1.6	104.9
193	—	27	0.128	0.09	1.2	19.8	—
240	0.37	13	0.128	0.076	0.539	47.9	—
570	0.79	37	0.14	0.096	1.04	10.1	—
—	—	0	0.274	0.108	0.632	0.7	—
—	—	16	0.26	0.155	1.25	17	—
163	0.15	141	0.082	0.207	0.755	62.8	68.4
246	0.18	13	0.05	0.03	0.3	47.3	56.7
227	0.3	2455	0.034	0.056	0.506	2.3	13.9
136	2.6	302	.014	.351	.118	0	20
187	2.38	252	.028	.488	.63	0	62
188	3.75	253	.037	.389	.082	0	16
62	2.88	—	—	—	—	0	—
120	3.9	174	.03	.334	.063	0	21
81	—	—	.06	.279	106	0	10
128	2.10	—	.08	.503	.158	0	58

food	water	energy	pro-tein	fat	carbo-hydrate	cal-cium	phos-phorus	iron
	%	kcal	←——————— gm ———————→			←————————————— mg		
Muenster	41.77	368	23.41	30.04	1.12	717	468	.41
Parmesan,								
grated	17.66	456	41.56	30.02	3.74	1376	807	.95
Roquefort	39.38	369	21.54	30.64	2.	662	392	.56
Swiss	37.21	376	28.43	27.45	3.38	961	605	.17
goat's milk	87.03	69	3.56	4.14	4.45	134	111	.05
kale	91.2	32	1.9	0.4	5.63	72	28	0.9
lamb's-quarters	88.9	32	3.2	0.7	5.	258	45	0.7
mustard greens	94.46	15	2.26	0.24	2.1	74	41	0.7
mung sprouts								
raw	90.4	30	3.04	0.18	5.93	13	54	0.91
nuts								
almonds								
toasted, unblanched	2.6	589	20.38	50.77	22.91	283	550	4.92
cashews								
dry roasted	1.7	574	15.31	46.35	32.69	45	490	6.
pignolias (pinenuts)								
dried	6.69	515	24	50.7	14.22	26	508	9.2
pistachios								
dry roasted	2.09	606	14.93	52.82	27.53	70	476	3.17
onions	92.24	28	0.9	0.16	6.28	27	23	0.2
oranges	86.75	47	0.94	0.12	11.75	40	14	0.1
peanut butter	1.29	591	28.48	51.14	15.84	33	374	1.81
peanuts								
oil roasted	1.99	580	26.78	49.19	18.48	86	506	1.92
rose-apples								
raw	93	25	0.6	0.3	5.7	29	8	0.07
seeds								
pumpkin & squash								
whole, roasted	4.5	446	18.55	19.4	53.75	55	92	3.31
sesame								
whole, roasted	3.3	565	16.96	48	25.74	989	638	14.76
sunflower								
kernels, dried	5.36	570	22.78	49.57	18.76	116	705	6.77

potas-sium	zinc	vit. A	thiamin	ribo-flavin	niacin	vit. C	folacin
		RE	←———————————————— mg ————————————————→				mcg
134	2.81	316	.013	.32	.103	0	12
107	3.19	—	.045	.386	.315	0	8
91	2.08	—	.04	.586	.734	0	49
111	3.9	253	.022	.365	.092	0	6
204	.3	56	.048	.138	.277	1.29	1
228	0.24	740	0.053	0.07	0.5	41	13.3
—	—	970	0.1	0.26	0.9	37.	—
202	—	303	0.041	0.063	0.433	25.3	—
149	0.41	2	0.084	0.124	0.749	13.2	60.8
773	4.92	0	0.131	0.601	2.829	0.7	64.1
565	5.6	0	0.2	0.2	1.4	0	69.2
599	4.25	—	0.81	0.19	3.57	—	—
970	1.36	—	0.423	0.246	1.408	—	—
152	0.18	0	0.042	0.008	0.08	5.7	12.7
181	0.07	21	0.087	0.04	0.282	53.2	30.3
703	6.62	0	0.293	0.101	14.796	0	105.6
685	2.29	—	0.147	0.105	13.444	0	82.
123	0.06	34	0.02.	0.03	0.8	22.3	—
919	10.3	—	—	—	—	—	—
475	7.16	—	—	—	—	—	—
689	5.06	5	2.29	0.25	4.5	—	—

food	water	energy	pro-tein	fat	carbo-hydrate	cal-cium	phos-phorus	iron
	%	kcal	←———	gm	———→	←———		mg
squash								
summer, cooked	93.7	20	0.91	0.31	4.31	27	39	0.36
squash								
winter, baked	89.02	39	0.89	0.63	8.75	14	20	0.33
water chestnuts								
raw	73.46	106	1.4	0.1	23.94	11	615	0.6
yogurt								
skim milk	85.23	56	5.73	0.18	7.68	199	156	.09

Source: United States Department of Agriculture Handbooks, *Composition of Foods*, Series 8 (Washington, D.C.: U.S. Government Printing Office). No. 8-1, *Dairy and Egg Products*, 1976; No. 8-9, *Fruits and Fruit Juices*, 1982; No. 8-11, *Vegetables and Vegetable Products*, 1984; No. 8-12, *Nut and Seed Products*, 1984.

potas-sium	zinc	vit. A	thiamin	ribo-flavin	niacin	vit. C	folacin
→		RE	←		mg	→	mcg
192	0.39	29	0.044	0.041	0.513	5.5	20.1
437	0.26	356	0.085	0.024	0.701	9.6	28
584	—	0	0.14	0.2	1	4	—
255	.97	2	.048	.234	.124	.87	12

Limited Glossary

ADAPTOGEN: A substance that increases our ability to deal with the negative effects of stress (e.g., ginseng is used for such purposes in Russia).

ALLERGEN: A substance that brings about an allergic reaction.

ANTIBODY: Proteins produced by the body in response to an offending agent.

ANTIGEN: Any substance that brings about the production of antibodies. Antigens may be externally introduced or formed within the body.

AUTOANTIBODIES: A self-produced antibody acting against a person's own body.

AUTOANTIGENS: Any substance within our own body that brings about an antibody reaction.

CARCINOGEN: An agent that causes cancer.

CELL-MEDIATED IMMUNITY: Types of immune reactions that involve T cells.

CYTOTOXIN: A poison that attacks various tissues and organs and is produced by introducing foreign cells.

FREE RADICAL: A molecular fragment that is capable of damaging the cells, producing genetic damage, and perhaps even causing cancer.

HOMEOPATHIC: A type of drugless therapy based on the theory of "like cures like"; opposite of *allopathy,* where drugs are used.

HUMORAL IMMUNITY: Various immune-related substances and actions generated by the bodily fluids.

INTERFERONS: The first line of defense against invading viruses; they are proteins made by our cells under viral attack and serve to inhibit the multiplication of a broad range of viruses.

LYMPHOCYTE: A type of white blood cell without certain granules; it numbers from 25 to 30 percent of total white cells in normal individuals. (Note: throughout this book, to minimize confusion, *lymphocyte* and *white blood cell* have been used interchangeably.)

MACROPHAGE: A cell able to engulf foreign particulate substances.

MICROBE: A micro-organism (e.g., bacterium, fungus, virus, protozoan).

MICRONUTRIENT: A nutrient needed by the body in extremely *small* quantities (e.g., we need calcium in *large* quantities, and it is called a *macronutrient*).

MUTAGEN: An agent able to induce cell mutation, a step along the cancer process.

NATURAL KILLER CELLS: NK cells recognize and kill invaders *without* any known antigenic stimulation and without any antibody to the invaders.

PHAGOCYTES: Cells that kill, remove, and dispose of invading microbes.

PHAGOCYTOSIS: The engulfing of particles by single cells.

T AND B CELLS: White cells, derived from the thymus gland and bone marrow, respectively.

T HELPER CELLS: White cells that attack an invading organism.

T SUPPRESSOR CELLS: White cells that stop the action of T helper cells once the invaders have been destroyed; when T suppressor cells increase disproportionately in number, they may destroy our ability to fight infection, hence destroying our immune system.

T HELPER TO T SUPPRESSOR RATIO: The ratio of T helper to T suppressor cells, normally about 1.8:1 in healthy individuals. (See Appendix 1 for ratios in disease states.)

References*

Abbassy, A. S., et al. (1974). Studies of cell-mediated immunity and allergy in protein energy malnutrition. *Am. J. Trop. Med. Hyg.* 77: 18–21.

Ackerman, L. V. (1972). Some thoughts on nutrition and cancer. *Nutrition and Cancer* 1: 2–8.

Adams, J. (1978). Improving stress management. *Social Change* 8: 1–12.

Ader, R., ed. (1981). *Psychoneuroimmunology.* Academic Press, N.Y.

Ader, R., and Cohen, N. (1975). Behaviorally conditioned immunosuppression. *Psychosom. Med.* 37: 333.

———. (1981). Conditioned immunopharmacologic responses, in *Psychoneuroimmunology,* Ader, R., ed. Academic Press, N.Y.

Agnello, V. (1978). Complement deficiency states. *Medicine* 57: 1–23.

Ahlqvist, J. (1981). Hormonal influences on immunologic and related phenomena, in *Psychoneuroimmunology,* Ader, R., ed., Academic Press, N.Y.

Akhtar, H. (1984). Kaposi's sarcoma in renal transplant recipients. *Cancer* 53(2): 258–266.

Alderson, R. M. (1981). Nutrition and cancer: evidence from epidemiology. *Proc. Nutr. Soc.* 40: 1.

Aleksandrowicz, J., et al. (1977). Effects of food enrichment with various doses of selenium selenate on some immune responses in laboratory animals. *Rocz. Nauk. Zootech.* 4: 113–126.

Allington, H. V., and Allington, R. R. (1954). Insect bites. *J. Am. Med. Assoc.* 155: 240–247.

Allison, A. C. (1974). The roles of T and B lymphocytes in self-tolerance and autoimmunity. *Contemp. Top. Immunobiol.* 3: 227.

Alper, C. A.; Colten, H. R.; and Rosen, F. S. (1972). Homozygous deficiency of C_3 in a patient with repeated infection. *Lancet* 2: 1179–1181.

---

*While the references are intended to guide the interested reader to original sources, complete citations are not always given.

Ames, B. N.; McCann, J.; and Yamasaki, E. (1975). Methods for detecting carcinogens. *Mutat. Res.* 31: 347.

Amkraut, A. A., and Solomon, G. F. (1975). From the symbolic stimulus to the pathophysiologic response: immune mechanisms. *Int. J. Psychiatry Med.* 5: 541–563.

Anderson, D. D.; Deckert, T.; and Nerup, J., eds. (1975). *Immunological Aspects of Diabetes Mellitus.* Gentofte Acta Endocrinol., Copenhagen.

Anderson, J. R.; Buchanan, W. W.; and Goudie, R. B. (1967). *Autoimmunity, Clinical and Experimental.* Charles C. Thomas, Springfield, Ill.

Anonymous (1977). *Smoking or Health. Third Report of the Royal College of Physicians.* Pitman Medical Publishing Co., Ltd., London.

———. (1979). The effect of oral contraceptives on blood vitamin A levels and the role of sex hormones. *Nutrition Reviews* 37: 346–348.

———. (1981). Fat-soluble vitamin nutrition in patients with chronic renal disease. *Nutrition Reviews* 39: 212–214.

———. (1982a). Coffee consumption and cancer of the pancreas. *Nutrition Reviews* 40: 262–263.

———. (1982b). Dietary carotene and the risk of lung cancer. *Nutrition Reviews* 40: 265–268.

———. (1984). Update: AIDS-United States. *Morbidity and Mortality Weekly Report* 33: 337–339 (June 22, 1984).

Aoki, S.; Ikuta, K.; and Aoyama, G. (1972). Induction of chronic polyarthritis in rabbits. *Nature* 237: 168–169.

Arbesman, C. E., et al. (1966). The allergic response to stinging insects VII. Extracts of yellow jacket. *J. Allergy* 38: 1–7.

———. (1965). The allergic response of stinging insects IV. Cross reactions between bee, wasp, and yellow jacket. *J. Allergy* 37: 147–157.

Aref, G. H.; El-Din, M. K.; and Hassan, A. J. (1970). Immunoglobulins in kwashiorkor. *Am. J. Trop. Med. Hyg.* 73: 186–191.

Arky, R. A. (1983). Prevention and therapy of diabetes mellitus. *Nutrition Reviews* 6: 165–170.

Asp, N. G., et al. (1979). Dietary fibre and experimental colon cancer in the rat. *Nutrition and Cancer* 1: 70.

Austen, K. F. (1978). Homeostasis of effector systems which can also be recruited for immunologic reactions. Presidential Address, American Association of Immunologists, Atlanta, Ga.

———. (1977). Introduction to clinical immunology, in *Harrison's Principles of Internal Medicine,* Thorn, G. W., et al., eds., McGraw-Hill Book Co., N.Y.

Austin, F. G. (1974). Schistosoma mansoni chemoprophylaxis with dietary lapachol. *Am. J. Trop. Med. Hyg.* 23: 412–415.

Axelrod, A. E. (1971). Immune processes in vitamin deficiency states. *Am. J. Clin. Nutr.* 24: 265–271.

Bach, J. F., et al. (1972). Evidence for a serum factor secreted by the human thymus. *Lancet* 2: 1056.

Bach, M., and Bach, J. (1981). Imbalance in T cell subsets in human diseases. *Int. J. Immunopharmac.* 3: 269–273.

Bach, M. A., et al. (1981). Studies on T cell subsets and functions in leprosy. *Clin. Exp. Immun.* 44: 491–500.

———. (1980). Deficit of suppressor T cells in active multiple sclerosis. *Lancet* 2: 1221–1224.

Baggs, R. B., and Miller, S. A. (1974). Defect in resistance to Salmonella typhimurium in iron-deficient rats. *J. Infect. Diseases* 130: 409–411.

———. (1973). Nutritional iron deficiency as a determinant of host resistance in the rat. *J. Nutr.* 103: 1554–1560.

Bahrke, M. S. (1981). Alterations in anxiety following exercise and rest, in *Exercise in Health and Disease,* Nagle, F. J. and Montoye, eds., Charles C. Thomas, Springfield, Ill.

Baker, H. (1983). Analysis of vitamin status. *J. Med. Soc. N.J.* 80 (8): 633–636.

Ballentine, R. (1978). *Diet and Nutrition.* Himalayan International Institute, Honesdale, Pa.

Bang, B. G., et al. (1975). T and B lymphocyte rosetting in undernourished children. *Proc. Soc. Exp. Biol. Med.* 149: 199–202.

Barbosa, J., et al. (1980). Linkage analysis between the major histocompatibility system and insulin-dependent diabetes in families with patients in two consecutive generations. *J. Clin. Invest.* 65: 592–601.

———. (1978). Analysis of linkage between the major histocompatibility system and juvenile, insulin-dependent diabetes in multiplex families: reanalysis of data. *J. Clin. Invest.* 62: 492–495.

Barnett, A. H., et al. (1981). Diabetes in identical twins: a study of 200 pairs. *Diabetologia* 20: 87–93.

Barr, S. E. (1971). Allergy to hymenoptera stings — review of the world literature: 1953–1970. *Ann. Allergy* 29: 49–66.

———. (1967). Allergy to insect stings: clinical and laboratory studies. *Med. Ann. D. C.* 36: 395.

Barrett, J. T. (1980). *Basic Immunology and Its Medical Application.* C. V. Mosby Co., St. Louis.

Barrios, B. A., and Shigetomi, C. C. (1980). Coping-skills training: potential for prevention of fears and anxieties. *Behavior Therapy* 11: 431–439.

———. (1979). Coping-skills training for the management of anxiety: a critical review. *Behavior Therapy* 10: 491–522.

Barthrop, R., et al. (1977). Depressed lymphocyte function after bereavement. *Lancet* 1: 834.

Bass, D. A., et al. (1977). Polymorphonuclear leukocyte bactericidal activity and oxidative metabolism during glutathione peroxidase deficiency. *Infect. Immun.* 18: 78–84.

Bauernfiend, J. C. (1981). *Carotenoids as Colorants and Vitamin A Precursors.* Academic Press, N.Y.

Bauernfiend, J. C., and Pinkert, D. M. (1970). Food processing with added ascorbic acid. *Adv. Food Res.* 18: 219.

Baugh, A., et al. (1965). Studies on hypersensitivity to hymenoptera I. antigenicity and cross reactivity of body extracts. *Ann. Allergy* 23: 430–433.

Baumbartner, W. A.; Hill, V. A.; and Wright, E. T. (1978). Antioxidant effects in the development of Ehrlich ascites carcinoma. *Am. J. Clin. Nutr.* 31: 457–465.

Beach, R. S.; Gershwin, M. E.; and Hurley L. S. (1982). Zinc, copper, and manganese in immune function and experimental oncogenesis. *Nutrition and Cancer* 3: 172–191.

Beisel, W. R. (1977). Malnutrition as a consequence of stress, in *Malnutrition and the Immune Response,* Suskind, R. M., ed., Raven Press, N.Y.

———. (1979). Malnutrition and the immune response, in *Biochemistry of Nutrition I.,* Neuberger, A., and Jukes, T. H., eds., University Park Press, Baltimore.

———. (1982). Single nutrients and immunity. *Am. J. Clin. Nutr.* 35: 417–468.

Beisel, W. R.; Edelman, R.; Nauss, K.; and Suskind, R. M. (1981). Single-nutrient effects on immunologic functions. *J. Am. Med. Assoc.* 245: 53–58.

Bell, R. G., et al. (1976). Serum and small intestinal immunoglobulin levels in under-nourished children. *Am. J. Clin. Nutr.* 29: 392–397.

Bender, A. E. (1982). Diet and killer diseases — evidence or opinion? in *Nutrition and Killer Diseases,* Rose, J., ed., Noyes Publications, Park Ridge, N.J.

Bennett, J. C. (1978). The infectious etiology of rheumatoid arthritis: new considerations. *Arthritis Rheum.* 62: 12–30.

Benson, H. (1975). *The Relaxation Response.* William Morrow, N.Y.

Berenstein, T. F. (1972). Effect of selenium and vitamin E on antibody formation in rabbits. *Zdravookhr Beloruss* 18: 74–76.

Berg, J. W.; Howell, M. A.; and Silverman, S. J. (1973). Dietary hypotheses and diet-related research in the etiology of colon cancer. *Health Service Report* 88: 915–924.

Berger, M., and Berchtold, P. (1977). The role of physical exercise and training in the management of diabetes mellitus. *Bibliotheca Nutritio et Dieta.* 27.

Bergsma, D., and Good, R. A., eds. (1968). *Immunological Deficiency Diseases in Man,* National Foundation — March of Dimes Original Article Series, National Foundation, N.Y.

Bergsma, D.; Good, R. A.; and Finstad, J., eds. (1975). *Immunodeficiency in Man and Animals,* National Foundation — March of Dimes Original Article Series, Sinauer Associates, Sunderland, Mass.

Bernauer, W. N. (1980). *The Use of Hypnosis in the Treatment of Cancer Patients: A Five Year Report.* ASCH Annual Scientific Program, Los Angeles.

Bernheim, H. A.; Block, L. H.; and Atkins, E. (1979). Fever: pathogenesis, pathophysiology, and purpose. *Annals Int. Med.* 91: 261–270.

Bernstein, D., and Borkovec, T. (1973). *Progressive Relaxation Training.* Research Press, Champaign, Ill.

Bernstein, D. S., et al. (1966). Prevalence of osteoporosis in high- and low-fluoride areas in North Dakota. *J. Am. Med. Assoc.* 198: 499.

Bernton, H. S., and Brown, H. (1964). Insect allergy — preliminary studies of the cockroach. *J. Allergy* 35: 506.

Bersani, G., et al. (1981). Lymphocyte subpopulations in insulin-dependent diabetics with and without serum islet-cell antibodies. *Diabetologia* 20: 47–50.

Besedovsky, H. O., and Sorkin, E. (1981). Immunologic-neuroendocrine circuits: physiological approaches, in *Psychoneuroimmunology,* Ader, R., ed., Academic Press, N.Y.

Best, E. W. R.; Josie, G. H.; and Walker, C. B. (1961). A Canadian study of mortality in relation to smoking habits: a preliminary report. *Can. J. Public Health* 52: 99–106.

Bigazzi, P. E., and Rose, N. R. (1975). Spontaneous autoimmune thyroiditis in animals as a model for human disease. *Prog. Allergy* 19: 245.

Binder, C., and Faber, O. K. (1978). Residual beta-cell function and its metabolic consequences. *Diabetes* 28: supplement 1: 226–229.

Binderup, L.; Bramm, E.; and Arrigoni-Martelli, E. (1980). Effect of D-penicillamine in vitro and in vivo on macrophage phagocytosis. *Biochem. Pharmacol.* 29: 2273–2278.

Bland, J. (1984). "Hidden" diseases caused by candida. *Prev. Med.* 3 (4): 12.

Blomgren, H., et al. (1978). Evidence for the appearance of nonspecific suppressor cells in the blood after local radiation therapy. *Int. J. Radiat. Oncol. Biol. Phys.* 4: 249–253.

Bluestein, H. G.; Williams, G. W.; and Steinberg, A. D. (1981). Cerebrospinal fluid antibodies to neuronal cells: association with neuropsychiatric manifestations of systemic lupus erythematosus. *J. Am. Med. Assoc.* 70: 240–246.

Blumenthal, J. A., et al. (1982). Psychological changes accompany aerobic exercise in healthy middle-aged adults. *Psychosom. Med.* 44: 529–536.

Bois, P. (1963). Effect of magnesium deficiency on mast cells and urinary histamine in rats. *Br. Exp. Pathol.* 44: 151–155.

Bollag, W. (1983). Vitamin A and retinoids. *Lancet* April 16, 1983, 860.

Bottazzo, G. F., and Doniach, D. (1978). Islet-cell antibodies in diabetes mellitus: evidence of an autoantigen common to all cells in the islet of Langerhans. *Ric. Clin. Lab.* 8: 29–38.

Bottazzo, G. F.; Florin-Christensen, A.; and Doniach, D. (1974). Islet-cell antibodies in diabetes mellitus with autoimmune polyendocrine deficiencies. *Lancet* 2: 1279–1283.

Boyd, E. (1932). The weight of the thymus gland in health and in disease. *Am. J. Dis. Child* 42: 116.

Boyd, W. C. (1966). *Fundamentals of Immunology.* Interscience Publishers, N.Y.

Boyne, R., and Arthur, J. R. (1979). Alterations of neutrophil functions in deficient cattle. *J. Comp. Pathol.* 89: 151–158.

Brinton, L. A., et al. (1979). Breast cancer risk factors among screening program participants. *J. Natl. Cancer Inst.* 62: 34–44.

Brown, D. G., and Burk, R. F. (1973). Selenium retention in tissues and sperm of rats fed a torula yeast diet. *J. Nutr.* 103: 102–108.

Brown, R. E., and Katz, M. (1966a). Failure of antibody production to yellow fever vaccine in children with kwashiorkor. *Trop. Geogr. Med.* 18: 125–128.

———. (1966b). Smallpox vaccination in malnourished children. *Trop. Geogr. Med.* 18: 129–132.

Bruton, O. C. (1952). Agammaglobulinemia. *Pediatrics* 9: 722–728.

Buchanan, N., et al. (1973). Urinary tract infection and secretory urinary IgA in malnutrition. *S. Afr. Med. J.* 47: 1179–1181.

Buckley, C. E., and Dorsey, F. C. (1970). The effect of aging on human serum immunoglobulin concentrations. *J. Immunol.* 105: 964–972.

Buckley, R. H. (1975). Iron deficiency anemia: in relationship to infection susceptibility and host defense. *J. Pediatr.* 86: 993–995.

———. (1980). Disorders of the IgE System, in *Immunologic Disorders in Infants and Children,* Steihm, E. R., and Fulginiti, V. A., eds., W. B. Saunders, Philadelphia.

Burk, R. F. (1976). Selenium in man, in *Trace Elements in Human Health and Disease,* Prasad, A., ed., Academic Press, N.Y.

Burkitt, D. P. (1971). Epidemiology of cancer of the colon and rectum. *Cancer* 28: 3–13.

Burnet, M. (1972). *Auto-Immunity and Auto-Immune Disease.* F. A. Davis Co., Philadelphia.

Busse, W. W., et al. (1975). Immunotherapy in bee sting anaphylaxis. Use of honey bee venom. *J. Am. Med. Assoc.* 231: 1154–1156.

CDC. (1984). Update: AIDS — United States. *MMWR* 33: 688–691.

———. (1985a). Update: AIDS — Europe. *MMWR* 34: 147–150.

———. (1985b). Update: AIDS — United States. *MMWR* 34: 245–248.

Cahill, G. F., and McDevitt, H. O. (1981). Insulin-dependent diabetes mellitus: the initial lesion. *N. Engl. J. Med.* 304: 1454–1465.

Cameron, E., and Pauling, L. (1980). On cancer and vitamin C. *Executive Health* 16: 4.

Cantwell, J. D. (1978). Running. *J. Am. Med. Assoc.* 240: 1409–1410.

Carlsson, B., et al. (1976). Escherichia coli O antibody content in milk from healthy Swedish mothers and mothers from a very low socio-economic group of a developing country. *Acta Pediat. Scand.* 65: 417–423.

Carroll, K. K. (1975). Experimental evidence of dietary factors and hormone-dependent cancers. *Cancer Res.* 35: 3374–3383.

———. (1977). Dietary factors in hormone-dependent cancers, in *Nutrition and Cancer,* Winick, M., ed., John Wiley & Sons, N.Y.

Cassell, J. (1970). Physical illness in response to stress, in *Social Stress,* Levine, S., and Scotch, N., eds., Aldine, Chicago.

Cathcart, R. F. (1975). Clinical trial of vitamin C. *Med. Tribune,* June 25.

———. (1981). Vitamin C, titrating to bowel tolerance, anascorbemia, and acute induced scurvey. *Med. Hypotheses* 7: 1359–1376.

———. (1984). Vitamin C in the treatment of acquired immune deficiency syndrome (AIDS). *Med. Hypotheses* 14: 423–433.

Chandra, R. K. (1972). Immunocompetence in undernutrition. *J. Pediatr.* 81: 1194–1200.

———. (1974). Rosette-forming T lymphocytes and cell-mediated immunity in malnutrition. *Brit. Med. J.* 545: 608–609.

———. (1975a). Food antibodies in malnutrition. *Arch. Dis. Child.* 50: 532–534.

———. (1975b). Reduced secretory antibody response to live attenuated measles and poliovirus vaccines in malnourished children. *Brit. Med. J.* 2: 583–585.

———. (1975c). Serum complement and immunoconglutinin in malnutrition. *Arch. Dis. Child.* 50: 225–229.

———. (1977). Lymphocyte subpopulations in human malnutrition: cytotoxic and suppressor cells. *Pediatrics* 59: 423–427.

————. (1980a). *Immunology of Nutritional Disorders.* Edward Arnold, Chicago, Ill.

————. (1980b). Symposium: nutritional deficiency, immune responses, and infectious illness. *Fed. Proc.* 39: 3086.

————. (1981). Immunocompetence as a functional index of nutritional status. *Brit. Med. Bul.* 37: 89–94.

Chandra, R. K., and Newberne, P. M. (1977). *Nutrition, Immunity and Infection: Mechanisms of Interaction.* Plenum Press, N.Y.

Chang, S. S., and Rasmussen, A. F. (1965). Stress-induced suppression of interferon production in virus infected mice. *Nature* 205: 623–625.

Chang, W. W. Y. (1980). Pollen survey of the United States, in *Allergic Diseases,* Patterson, R., ed., J. B. Lippincott Co., Philadelphia.

Chatenoud, L., et al. (1980). Deficiency of suppressor/cytotoxic T cells in idiopathic membranous glomerulonephritis. *Immun. Letts.* 2: 167–168.

Chen, J. R., and Anderson, J. M. (1979). Legionnaire's disease: concentrations of selenium and other elements. *Science* 206: 1426–1427.

Chen, W. Y., et al. (1961). Site distribution of cancer deaths in husband-wife and sibling pairs. *JNCI* 27: 875.

Christau B., et al. (1977). Incidence, seasonal and geographic patterns of juvenile-onset insulin-dependent diabetes mellitus in Denmark. *Diabetologia* 13: 281–284.

Chu, E. W., and Malmgren, R. A. (1965). An inhibitory effect of vitamin A on the induction of tumors of forestomach and cervix in the Syrian hamster by polycyclic hydrocarbons. *Cancer Res.* 23: 884–895.

Church, C. F., and Church, H. N. (1975). *Food Values of Portions Commonly Used.* J. B. Lippincott Co., Philadelphia.

Clark, L. C.; Graham, G. F.; Crounse, R. G.; Grimson, R.; Hulka, B.; and Shy, C. M. (1984). Plasma selenium and skin neoplasms: a case-control study. *Nutrition and Cancer* 6 (1): 13–18.

Clausen, J. P. (1977). Effect of physical training on cardiovascular adjustments to exercise in man. *Physiol. Rev.* 57: 779–816.

Cline, M. J. (1975). *The White Cell.* Harvard University Press, Cambridge.

Clumeck, Nathan, et al. (1984). Acquired immunodeficiency syndrome in African patients. *N. Engl. J. Med.* 310: 492–497.

Cohen, B. E., and Cohen, I. K. (1973). Vitamin A: adjuvant and steroid antagonist in the immune response. *J. Immunol.* 3: 1376–1380.

Cooke, A., and Lydyard, P. M. (1980). The role of T cells in autoimmune disease. *Path. Res. Prac.* 1: 70.

Coombs, R. R. A., and Gell, P. G. H., eds. (1968). *Clinical Aspects of Immunology.* F. A. Davis Co., Philadelphia.

Cox, F. E. G. (1984). How parasites evade the immune response. *Immunology Today* 5 (2): 29.

Craighead, J. E. (1978). Current views on the etiology of insulin-dependent diabetes mellitus. *N. Engl. J. Med.* 299: 1439–1445.

Crary, E. J.; Smyrna, G.; and McCarty, M. F. (1984). Potential applications for high-dose nutritional antioxidants. *Med. Hypotheses* 13: 77–98.

Creutzfeldt, W.; Kobberling, J.; and Neel, J. V., eds. (1976). *The Genetics of Diabetes Mellitus.* Springer-Verlag, Berlin.

Cruse, P.; Lewin, M.; and Clark, C. G. (1979). Dietary cholesterol is cocarcinogenic for human colon cancer. *Lancet* 1: 752–755.

Cudworth, A. G. (1978). Type I diabetes mellitus. *Diabetologia* 14: 281–291.

Cudworth, A. G., and Festenstein, H. (1978). HLA genetic heterogeneity in diabetes mellitus. *Brit. Med. Bul.* 34: 285–289.

Cunningham, A. J. (1978). *Understanding Immunology.* Academic Press, N.Y.

———. (1981). Mind, body and immune response, in *Psychoneuroimmunology,* Ader, R., ed., Academic Press, N.Y.

Cunningham, A. S. (1976). Lymphomas and animal-protein consumption. *Lancet* 2: 1184–1186.

Cusick, M., et al. (1979). Malaria surveillance and control in Sutter-Yuba counties. *J. Calif. Morbidity* 49:

Cutler, S. J., and Young, J. L., eds. (1975). The third national cancer survey: incidence data. *Natl. Cancer Inst. Monogr.* 41: 1–454.

Da Prato, R. (1984). Fatty acid-ion exchange complexes in the treatment of candida albicans. *Ecological Formulas* 1: 5–6.

Davis, C. (1979). *Insects, Allergy and Disease.* Davis Publications, the Miracle Press, Ltd., Ottawa, Ontario, Canada.

Dawber, T. R.; Meadors, G. P.; and Moore, F. E. (1951). Epidemiological approaches to heart disease: Framingham study. *Am. J. Public Health* 41: 279–286.

Dayton, S., et al. (1969). A controlled chemical trial of a diet high in unsaturated fat in preventing complications of atherosclerosis. *Circulation* 39–40, supplement 2: 1–63.

Decker, T. W.; Williams, J. M.; and Hall, D. (1982). Preventive training in management of stress for reduction of physiological symptoms through increased cognitive and behavioral controls. *Psychological Reports* 50: 1327–1334.

DeJong, U. W., et al. (1974). Aetiological factors in oesophageal cancer in Singapore Chinese. *Int. J. Cancer* 13: 291–303.

DeLuca, H. F. (1977). Vitamin D metabolism. *Clin. Endoc.* 7: 1.

DeLuca, L., et al. (1972). Maintenance of epithelial cell differentiation: the mode of action of vitamin A. *Cancer* 30: 1331.

Denman, A. M. (1969). Anti-lymphocyte antibody and autoimmune disease; a review. *Clin. Exp. Immun.* 5: 217.

Deschamps, I., et al. (1980). HLA genotype studies in juvenile insulin-dependent diabetes. *Diabetologia* 19: 189–193.

Desowitz, R. S., and Barnwell, J. W. (1980). Effect of selenium and dimethyl dioctadecyl ammonium bromide on the vaccine-induced immunity of Swiss-Webster mice against malaria (Plasmondium berghei). *Infect. Immun.* 27: 87–89.

De Swarte, R. D. (1980). Drug allergy, in *Allergic Diseases,* Patterson, R., ed., J. B. Lippincott Co., Philadelphia.

Detels, R., et al. (1983). Relation between sexual practices and T-cell subsets in homosexually active men. *Lancet* 1: 609–611.

Devesa, S. S., and Silverman, D. T. (1978). Cancer incidence and mortality trends in the United States. *J. Natl. Cancer Inst.* 60: 545–571.

deWaard, F. (1975). Breast cancer incidence and nutritional status with particular reference to body weight and height. *Cancer Res.* 35: 3351–3356.

———. (1982). Nutritional etiology of breast cancer: where are we now, and where are we going? *Nutrition and Cancer* 4: 85–89.

Diamond, H. S. (1982). Collagen autoimmune diseases, in *Handbook of Immunology for Students and House Staff.*

di Mario, U., et al. (1980). Immune complexes, islet-cell antibodies, antivirus antibodies, insulin antibodies, and HLA in insulin-dependent diabetes at diagnosis and follow-up. *Diabetologia* 19: 269.

Dobersen, M. J., et al. (1980). Cytotoxic autoantibodies to beta cells in the serum of patients with insulin-dependent diabetes mellitus. *N. Engl. J. Med.* 303: 1493–1498.

Doggert, D., et al. (1981). Cellular and molecular aspects of immune system aging. *Mol. Cell. Biochem.* 37: 156.

Doll, R. (1969). The geographical distribution of cancer. *Brit. J. Cancer* 1: 8.

Doll, R., and Peto, R. (1981). The causes of cancer: quantitative estimates of avoidable risks of cancer in the United States today. *J. Nat. Cancer Inst.* 66: 1191–1308.

Doniach, D. (1972). Autoimmunity in liver disease. *Prog. Clin. Immun.* 1: 45.

Doniach, D., Botazzo, G. F.; and Russell, R. C. G. (1979). Goitrous autoimmune thyroiditis (Hashimoto's disease), in *Clinics in Endocrinology and Metabolism,* Eversol, D., and Hall, R., eds., W. B. Saunders, London.

Dreizen, S. (1978). Nutrition and the immune response — a review. *Int. J. Vitam. Nutr. Res.* 49: 220–228.

Dubois, E. L., ed. (1974). *Lupus Erythematosus.* McGraw-Hill Book Co., N.Y.

Dujovne, C. A., and Azarnoff, D. L. (1973). Clinical complications of corticosteroid therapy: a selected review. *Med. Clin. N. Am.* 57: 1331.

Dumonde, D. C. (1966). Tissue-specific antigens. *Adv. Immun.* 5: 245.

Dyer, A. R., et al. (1975). High blood pressure: a risk factor for cancer mortality? *Lancet* 1: 1051–1056.

Eagle, R. (1981). *Eating and Allergy.* Doubleday & Co., Inc., N.Y.

Eastwood, M. A., et al. (1974). Perspectives on the bran hypothesis. *Lancet* 1: 1029–1033.

Edelman, R. (1977). Cell-mediated immune response in PCM — a review, in *Malnutrition and the Immune Response,* Suskind, R. M., ed., Raven Press, N.Y.

Ederer F., et al. (1971). Cancer among men on cholesterol-lowering diets: experience from five clinical trials. *Lancet* 2: 203–206.

Edwards, E., and Dean, L. (1977). Effects of crowding of mice and humoral antibody formation and protection to lethal antigenic challenge. *Psychosom. Med.* 39: 19.

Eggleston, D. W. (1984). Effect of dental amalgam and nickel alloys on T-lymphocytes: preliminary report. *J. Prosthetic Dentistry.* May 1984, 617–621.

Ehrenreich, B. A., and Cohn, Z. A. (1967). The uptake and digestion of iodinated human serum albumin by macrophages in vitro. *J. Exp. Med.* 126: 941–957.

Eisenbarth, G. S.; Morris, M. A.; and Scearce, R. M. (1981). Cytotoxic antibodies to cloned rat islet-cells in serum of patients with diabetes mellitus. *J. Clin. Invest.* 67: 403–408.

Eisenbarth, G. S., et al. (1980). Production of monoclonal antibodies reacting with peripheral blood mononuclear cell surface differentiation antigens. *J. Immunol.* 124: 1237–1244.

El-Hagrassy, M. M. O.; Banatvala, J. E.; and Coltart, D. J. (1980). Coxsackie-B-virus-specific IgM responses in patients with cardiac and other diseases. *Lancet* 2: 1160–1162.

Enck, R. E. (1979). Cancer in married couples. *Milty Med.* 144: 603.

Enig, M. G.; Munn, R. J.; and Keeney, M. (1978). Dietary fat and cancer trends — a critique. *Fed. Proc.* 37: 2215–2220.

Erickson, K. L., et al. (1980). Influence of dietary fat concentration and saturation on immune ontogeny in mice. *J. Nutr.* 110: 1555.

Fabris, N. (1973). Immunological reactivity during pregnancy in the mouse. *Experientia* 29: 610–612.

Fauman, M. A. (1982). The central nervous system and the immune system. *Biol. Psychiatry* 17: 1459–1482.

Fearon, D. T., and Austen, K. F. (1980). The alternate pathway of complement — a system of host resistance to microbial infection. *N. Engl. J. Med.* 303: 259–263.

Feinberg, A. R., and Feinberg, B. M. (1956). Asthma and rhinitis from insect allergens. *J. Allergy* 27: 437–444.

Feingold, B.; Benjamin, S. E.; and Michaeli, D. (1968). The allergic response to insect bites. *Ann. Rev. Entomol.* 13: 137–158.

Ferguson, A., and MacSween, R. N. M., eds. (1976). *Immunological Aspects of the Liver and Gastrointestinal Tract.* University Park Press, Baltimore.

Fernstrom, J. D. (1979). How food affects your brain. *Nutrition Action,* December 1979, 5–7.

Fialkow, P. J. (1969). Genetic aspects of autoimmunity. *Prog. Med. Gen.* 6: 117.

Fleckenstein, A. (1983). *Calcium Antagonism in Heart and Smooth Muscle.* John Wiley & Sons, N.Y.

Folkins, C. H., and Sime, W. E. (1981). Physical fitness training and mental health. *Am. Psychol.* 36: 373–389.

Food and Nutrition Board (1980). *Recommended Dietary Allowances.* National Academy of Sciences, Washington, D. C.

Ford, W. L. (1975). Lymphocyte migration and immune responses. *Prog. Allergy* 19: 1.

Forsham, P., et al. (1983). *Diabetes Forecast,* May-June, 23–26.

Fox, B. H. (1981). Psychosocial factors and the immune system in human cancer, in *Psychoneuroimmunology,* Ader, R., ed., Academic Press, N.Y.

Fox, S. M., and Haskell, W. L. (1978). Physical activity and the prevention of coronary heart disease. *NY Acad. Med. Bul.* 44: 950–965.

Frank, M. M., and Atkinson, J. P. (1975). Complement in clinical medicine. *Disease-a-Month,* January, 3–54.

Frank, M. M.; Gelfand, J. A.; and Atkinson, J. P. (1976). Hereditary angioedema: the clinical syndrome and management. *Annals Int. Med.* 84: 580–593.

Frankl, V. E. (1959). *From Death-Camp to Existentialism.* Beacon Press, Boston.

Frazier, C. A. (1965). Insect sting reactions in children. *Ann. Allergy* 23: 37–46.

———. (1966). Insect sting reactions in children — character, recognition, therapy. *Clin. Pediat.* 15: 463.

Freedman, S. O. (1971). *Clinical Immunology.* Harper & Row, Publishers, N.Y.

Friedman, M., and Rosenman, R. H. (1974). *Type A Behavior and Your Heart.* Knopf, N.Y.

Fudenberg, A. A., et al., eds. (1980). *Basic and Clinical Immunology.* Lange Medical Publishing, Los Altos.

Fudenberg, H. H. (1971). Are autoimmune diseases immunologic deficiency states? in *Immunobiology,* Good, R. A., and Fisher, D. W., eds., Sinauer Associates, Inc., Stamford, Conn.

Gamble, D. R. (1980). An epidemiological study of childhood diabetes affecting two or more siblings. *Diabetologia* 19: 341–344.

Gamble, D. R., and Taylor, K. W. (1969). Seasonal incidence of diabetes mellitus. *Brit. Med. J.* 3: 631–633.

Ganapathy, S. N., et al. (1977). Selenium content of selected foods, in *Trace Element Metabolism in Man and Animals,* Kirchgeber, M., ed., ATW, Freising-Weihenstephan, West Germany.

Ganda, O. P., and Soeldner, J. S. (1977). Genetic, acquired, and related factors in the etiology of diabetes mellitus. *Arch. Intern. Med.* 137: 461–469.

Garner, R. C. (1981). In vitro tests to detect chemical carcinogens. *Proc. Nutr. Soc.* 40: 75.

Garrison, J. E. (1978). Stress management training for the elderly: a psycho-educational approach. *J. Am. Geriatrics Soc.* 26: 397–403.

Gelernt, M. D., and Herbert, V. (1982). Mutagenicity of diisopropyla-mine dischloroacetate, the "active constituent" of vitamin B_{15} (pangamic acid). *Nutrition and Cancer* 3: 129–133.

Gelfand, E. W., and Desch, H. M., eds. (1980). *Biological Basis of Immuno-deficiency.* Raven Press, N.Y.

Gell, P. G. H.; Coombs, R. R. A.; and Lachmann, P. J., eds. (1975). *Clinical Aspects of Immunology,* 3rd ed. Blackwell Scientific Publications, Oxford.

Germann, D. R. (1977). *The Anti-Cancer Diet.* Wyden Books, Ridgefield, Conn.

Germuth, F. G., and Rodriguez, E. (1973). *Immunopathology of the Renal Glomerulus: Immune Complex Deposit and Antibasement Membrane Disease.* Little, Brown and Co., Boston.

Gerras, C., ed. (1976). *The Encyclopedia of Common Diseases.* Rodale Press, N.Y.

Gewurz, H. (1971). The immunologic role of complement, in *Immunobiology,* Good, R. A., and Fisher, D. W., eds., Sinauer Associates, Inc., Stamford, Conn.

Ginzler, E. M.; Bollet, A. J.; and Friedman, E. A. (1980). The natural history and response to therapy of lupus nephritis. *Ann. Rev. Med.* 31: 463–487.

Glynn, L. E., and Holborow, E. J. (1965). *Autoimmunity and Disease.* F. A. Davis Co., Philadelphia.

Golden, H. N., et al. (1978). Zinc and immunocompetence in protein energy malnutrition. *Lancet* 1: 1226-1228.

Good, R. A. (1981). Nutrition and immunity. *J. Clin. Immunol.* 1: 3.

Good, R. A.; Fernandez, G.; and Yunis, E. J. (1976). Nutritional deficiency, immunologic function and disease. *Am. J. Pathol.* 84: 599-614.

Gordon, G. (1983). New dimensions in calcium metabolism. *Osteopathic Annals* 11: 38-59.

Gottlieb, M. S., and Root, H. F. (1968). Diabetes mellitus in twins. *Diabetes* 17: 693-704.

Graham, S., and Mettlin, C. (1979). Diet and colon cancer. *Am. J. Epidemiol.* 109: 1-26.

Graham, S., et al. (1979). Genital cancer in wives of penile cancer patients. *Cancer* 44: 1870.

Greaves, M. F., and Janossy G. (1972). Elicitation of selective T and B lymphocyte responses by cell surface binding ligands. *Transplant Rev.* 11: 87-130.

Greenwood, E. D. (1976). Emotional well-being through exercise — therapeutic benefit for the adult, in *The Humanistic and Mental Health Aspects of Sports, Exercise and Recreation,* Craig, T. T., ed., American Medical Association, Chicago.

Gross, R. L., and Newberne, P. M. (1980). Role of nutrition in immunologic function. *Physiol. Rev.* 60: 188.

Guttler, F.; Seakins, J. W. T.; and Harkness, R. A., eds. (1979). *Inborn Errors of Immunity and Phagocytosis.* University Press, Baltimore.

Hafeman, D. G.; Sunde, R. A.; and Hoekstra, W. G. (1974). Effects of dietary selenium on erythrocyte and liver glutathione peroxidase in the rat. *J. Nutr.* 104: 580-586.

Hall, N. R., and Goldstein, A. L. (1981). Neurotransmitters and the immune system, in *Psychoneuroimmunology,* Ader, R., ed., Academic Press, N.Y.

Haller, O., et al. (1977). Role of non-conventional natural killer cells in resistance against syngeneic tumor cells in vivo. *Nature* 270: 609-611.

Hammond, E. C., and Horn, D. (1958). Smoking and death rates — report on 44 months of follow-up of 187,783 men. *J. Am. Med. Assoc.* 166: 1159-1172.

Hanson, L. A.; Ahlstedt, S.; et al. (1978). New knowledge in human milk immunoglobulin. *Acta Pediat. Scand.* 67: 577-582.

Hanson, L. A.; Carlsson, B.; et al. (1979). Immune response in the mammary gland, in *Immunology of Breast Milk,* Ogra, P. L., and Dayton, D., eds., Raven Press, N.Y.

Harber, L. C., and Baer, R. L. (1978). Reactions to light, heat and trauma, in *Immunological Diseases,* Amter, M., ed., Little, Brown and Co., Boston.

Harris, C., et al. (1983). Immunodeficiency among female sexual partners of males with acquired immunity deficiency syndrome (AIDS) — New York. *MMWR* 31: 697.

Hartung, G. H., and Farge, E. G. (1978). Personality and physiological traits in middle-aged runners and joggers. *J. Gerontol.* 32: 54–548.

Haurowitz, F. (1968). *Immunochemistry and the Biosynthesis of Antibodies.* Interscience Publishers, N.Y.

Hedfors, E.; Holm, G.; and Ohnell, B. (1976). Variations of blood lymphocytes during work. *Clin. Exp. Immun.* 24: 328–335.

Heidelberger, M. (1956). *Lectures in Immunochemistry.* Academic Press, N.Y.

Heiniger, H. J.; Brunner, K. T.; and Cerottini, J. C. (1978). Cholesterol: a critical cellular component for T lymphocyte cytotoxicity. *Proc. Natl. Acad. Sci. USA* 75: 568–576.

Hellstrom, K. E., and Hellstrom, I. (1971). Immunologic defenses against cancer, in *Immunobiology,* Good, R. A., and Fisher, D. W., eds., Sinauer Associates, Inc., Stamford, Conn.

Henry, J., and Stephens, P. (1977). *Stress, Health, and the Social Environment.* Springer-Verlag, N.Y.

Herbert, V. (1979). Pangamic acid (vitamin B_{15}). *Am. J. Clin. Nutr.* 32: 1534–1540.

———. (1980). *Nutrition Cultism: Facts and Fiction.* George F. Stickley Co., Philadelphia.

Herbert, V., and Barrett, S. (1981). *Vitamins and "Health" Foods: The Great American Hustle.* George F. Stickley Co., Philadelphia.

Hersko, C., et al. (1970). The effect of chronic iron deficiency on some biochemical functions of the human hematopoietic tissue. *Blood* 36: 321–327.

Higgs, D. J.; Morris, V. C.; and Levander, O. A. (1972). Effect of cooking on selenium content of foods. *J. Agric. Food Chem.* 20: 678.

Hill, M. J. (1979). Bacterial metabolism and colon cancer. *Nutr. Cancer* 1: 46.

———. (1981). Dietary fat and human cancer. *Proc. Nutr. Soc.* 40: 15.

Hill, M. J., et al. (1971). Bacteria and aetiology of cancer of large bowel. *Lancet* 1: 95–100.

Hinkle, L. (1957). The nature of man's adaptation to his total environment and the relationship of this to illness. *Arch. Intern. Med.* 99: 442.

Hinkle, L., et al. (1958). An investigation of the relation between life experience, personality characteristics, and general susceptibility to illness. *Psychosom. Med.* 20: 278.

Hirayama, T. (1967). *Smoking in Relation to the Death Rates of 265,118 Men and Women in Japan,* monograph, National Cancer Center, Research Institute, Tokyo.

Hirokawa, K., and Makinodan, T. (1975). Thymic involution: effect of T cell differentiation. *J. Immunol.* 114: 1661.

Hodes, H., and Kagen, B. M., eds. (1979). *Pediatric Immunology.* Science and Medicine Publishing, N.Y.

Hodges, R. E., et al. (1962). Factors affecting human antibody response: V. combined deficiencies of pantothenic acid and pyridoxine. *Am. J. Clin. Nutr.* 11: 187–199.

Holmes, T. H., and Rahe, R. H. (1967). The social readjustment rating scale. *Psychosom. Med.* 2: 213–218.

Horan, J. J., et al. (1977). Coping with pain: a component analysis of stress inoculation. *Cognitive Therapy and Res.* 1: 211–221.

Horowitz, S. D., and Hong, R. (1977). The pathogenesis and treatment of immunodeficiency. *Monogr. Allergy* 10: 1–198.

Horrobin, D. F., et al. (1979). The nutritional regulation of T lymphocyte function. *Med. Hypotheses* 5: 969–985.

Houghton, A., and Viola, M. (1981). Solar radiation and malignant melanoma of the skin. *Am. Acad. Derm.* 5: 477–482.

Huang, S. W., and Maclaren, N. K. (1976). Insulin-dependent diabetes: a disease of autoaggression. *Science* 192: 64–66.

Hume, D. M. (1971). Organ transplants and immunity, in *Immunobiology,* Good, R. A., and Fisher, D. W., eds., Sinauer Associates, Inc., Stamford, Conn.

Hunt, K. J., et al. (1978). A controlled trial of immunotherapy in insect hypersensitivity. *N. Engl. J. Med.* 299: 157–161.

Ikekawa, T., et al. (1969). Antitumor activity of aqueous extracts of edible mushrooms. *Cancer Res.* 29: 734–735.

Inman, R. D., and Day, N. K. (1981). Immunological and clinical aspects of immune complex disease. *Am. J. Med.* 70: 1097–1107.

Irvine, W. J. (1967). Immunobiology of the thymus and its relation to autoimmune disease. *Mod. Trends Immunnol.* 2: 250.

———, ed. (1980). *Immunology of Diabetes.* Teviot Scientific Publications, Edinburgh.

Ismail, A. H., and Young, R. G. (1973). The effect of chronic exercise on the personality of middle-aged men by univariate and multi-variate approaches. *J. Hum. Ergol.* 2: 47–57.

Jackson, G. (1960). The common cold. *Ann. Int. Med.* 53: 719.

Jackson, R. A., et al. (1982). Increased circulating Ia-antigen-bearing T cells in type I diabetes mellitus. *N. Engl. J. Med.* 306: 785–788.

Jacob-John, T. (1975). Oral polio vaccination of children in the tropics. *Am. J. Epidemiol.* 102: 414–421.

Jacobs, M. A. (1967). Interaction of psychologic and biologic predisposing factors in allergic disorders. *Psychosom. Med.* 29: 572.

Jacobs, M. A.; Spilken, A.; and Norman, M. (1969). Relationship of life change, maladaptive aggression and upper respiratory infection in male college students. *Psychosom. Med.* 31: 33–42.

James, G. V. (1982). Trace substances in foods and their effect on health, in *Nutrition and Killer Diseases,* Rose, J., ed., Noyes Publications, Park Ridge, N.J.

James, K., and Cullen, R. T. (1983). The effect of seminal plasma on macrophage function. *AIDS Research* 1 (1): 45–57.

Jee, W. S. S., et al. (1970). Corticosteroids and bone. *Am. J. Anat.* 129: 477.

Jenni, M. A., and Wollersheim, J. P. (1979). Cognitive therapy, stress management training, and the type A behavior pattern. *Cognitive Therapy and Res.* 3: 61–73.

Jenson, A. B.; Rosenberg, H. S.; and Notkins, A. L. (1980). Pancreatic islet-cell damage in children with fatal viral infections. *Lancet* 2: 354–358.

Jette, M. (1975). Habitual exercisers: a blood serum and personality profile. *J. Sports Med.* 3: 12–17.

Jick, H., and Dinan, B. J. (1981). Coffee and pancreatic cancer. *Lancet* 2: 92.

Johnson, F. C. (1971). Safety limits of phenolic antioxidants. *CRC Crit. Rev. Food Sci. Nutr.* 2: 267.

———. (1979). The antioxidant vitamins. *CRC Crit. Rev. Food Sci. Nutr.* 11: 217.

———. (1982). Carcinogenesis, vascular disease, and the free radical reaction. *Nutrition and Cancer* 3: 117–121.

———. (1983). Cancer promoters and initiators, and the free radical theory of carcinogenesis. *Nutrition and Cancer* 4: 169–170.

Johnson, P. M., and Faulk, W. P. (1976). Rheumatoid factor: its nature, specificity, and production in rheumatoid arthritis. *Clin. Immunol. Immunopathol.* 6: 414.

Johnson, T., et al. (1963). The influence of avoidance learning stress resistance to Coxsackie B virus. *J. Immunol.* 91: 569.

Jokl, E. (1977). The immunological status of athletes. *Medicine and Sport* 10.

Joossens, J. V., and Geboers, J. (1981). Nutrition and gastric cancer. *Proc. Nutr. Soc.* 40: 37.

Jowsey, J., et al. (1972). Effect of combined therapy with sodium fluoride, vitamin D and calcium in osteoporosis. *J. Am. Med. Assoc.* 53: 43.

Joynson, D. H. M., et al. (1972). Defect of cell-mediated immunity in patients with iron deficiency anaemia. *Lancet* 2: 1058-1059.

Kabat, E. A. (1968). *Structural Concepts in Immunology and Immunochemistry.* Holt, Rinehart & Winston, Inc., N.Y.

Kahn, H. A. (1966). The Dorn study of smoking and mortality among US veterans: report on 8½ years of observation. *Natl. Cancer Inst. Monogr.* 19: 1-125.

Kaplan, M. H. (1969). Autoimmunity to heart and its relation to heart disease; a review. *Prog. Allergy* 13: 408.

Kark, J. D., et al. (1982). Serum retinol and the inverse relationship between serum cholesterol and cancer. *Brit. Med. J.* 284: 152-154.

Katz, J., et al. (1969). Psychoendocrine considerations in cancer of the breast. *Ann. NY Acad. Sci.* 164: 509.

Katz, M., and Stiehm, E. R. (1977). Host defenses in malnutrition. *Pediatrics* 59: 490-495.

Kay, M. M. B. (1959). An overview of immune aging. *Mech. Aging Devel.* 9: 39-59.

Keet, M. P., and Thom, H. (1969). Serum immunoglobulins in kwashiorkor. *Arch. Dis. Child.* 44: 600-603.

Keeton, W. T. (1980). *Biological Science.* W. W. Norton & Co., N.Y.

Keller, S. E., et al. (1981). Suppression of immunity by stress: effect of a graded series of stressors on lymphocyte stimulation in the rat. *Psychosom. Med.* 43: 91.

Kelly, J. F., and Patterson, R. (1974). Anaphylaxis — course, mechanisms and treatment. *J. Am. Med. Assoc.* 227: 12.

Kessler, I. I. (1976). Human cervical cancer as a venereal disease. *Cancer Res.* 36: 783.

Kimber, D. C.; Gray, C. E.; Stackpole, C. E.; and Leavell, L. C. (1966). *Anatomy and Physiology* (15th ed.). Macmillan, N.Y.

Klayman, D. L. (1985). Qinghaosu (Artemisinin): an antimalarial drug from China. *Science* 228 (4703): 1049-1055.

Koch, W. F. (1961). *The Survival Factor in Neoplastic and Viral Diseases.* Vanderkloot Press, Inc.

Koller, L. D., et al. (1979). Synergism of methylmercury and selenium producing enhanced antibody formation in mice. *Arch. Environ. Health* 34: 248–251.

Kornfeld, H., et al. (1982). T-lymphocyte subpopulations in homosexual men. *N. Engl. J. Med.* 307: 729–731.

Krakauer, R. S., et al. (1979). Suppressor cell function defect in idiopathic systemic lupus erythematosus. *Clin. Immunol. Immunopathol.* 14: 327–333.

Kreitler, H., and Kreitler, S. (1970). Movement and aging: a psychological approach. *Medicine and Sport* 4: 302–306.

Kriebel, D., and Jowett, D. (1979). Stomach cancer mortality in north central states. *Nutr. Cancer* 1: 13.

Kyle, R. A., and Greipp, P. R. (1983). Multiple myeloma: houses and spouses. *Cancer* 51: 735.

Laake, H. (1960). The action of corticosteroids on the renal reabsorption of calcium. *Acta Endocr.* 34: 60.

Lahita, R., et al. (1979). Alterations of estrogen metabolism in SLE. *Arthritis Rheum.* 22: 1195.

Langer, E. L.; Janis, I. L.; and Wolfer, J. A. (1975). Reduction of psychological stress in surgical patients. *J. Exp. Soc. Psychol.* 11: 155–165.

Laube, H., and Pfeiffer, E. F. (1977). Exercise and diabetes mellitus. *Medicine and Sport* 10.

Layman, E. M. (1974). Psychological effects of physical activity, in *Exercise and Sports Sciences Reviews,* Whilmore, J. H., ed., Academic Press, N.Y.

Leaf, A. (1973). Unusual longevity: the common denominators. *Hospital Practice,* October 1973, 75–86.

Lepshitz, D. A., et al. (1971). The role of ascorbic acid in the metabolism of storage iron. *Brit. J. Haematol.* 20: 155–163.

Lernmark, A., et al. (1980). Antibodies directed against the pancreatic islet-cell plasma membrane: detection and specificity. *Diabetologia* 19: 445–451.

LeShan, L. (1977). *You Can Fight for Your Life.* M. Evans & Co., N.Y.

Lessof, M. H., ed. (1983). *Clinical Reactions to Food.* John Wiley & Sons, Chichester, England.

Levi, L. (1972). Stress and distress in response to psychosocial stimuli. *Acta Med. Scand.,* supplement: 528.

Levine, S. (1980). Tryptophan in biological psychiatry. *Orthomolecular Society Newsletter,* winter 1980.

Levitt, P. M., et al. (1979). *The Cancer Reference Book.* Paddington Press, Ltd., N.Y.

Levitt Research Laboratories, Inc. (1979). Anti-inflammatory compositions containing selenium compounds. *Chem. Abs.* 91: 96638s.

Levy, J. A., et al. (1982). Dietary fat affects immune response, production of antiviral factors and immune complex disease in NZB/NZW mice. *Proc. Natl. Acad. Sci. USA* 79: 1974.

Li, J. Y., et al. (1982). Correlation between cancers of the uterine cervix and penis in China. *JNCI* 69: 1063.

Lichtenstein, L. M.; Valentine, M. D.; and Sobotka, A. K. (1974). A case for venom treatment in anaphylactic sensitivity to hymenoptera stings. *N. Engl. J. Med.* 290: 1223.

Lin, R. S., and Kessler, I. (1981). A multifactorial model for pancreatic cancer in man: epidemiologic evidence. *J. Am. Med. Assoc.* 245: 147–152.

Littler, J. R. (1981). Anti-rheumatic drugs. *Pharmacol. Ther.* 15: 45–68.

Lloyd, N., and Schur, P. (1981). Immune complexes, complement, and anti-DNA in exacerbations of systemic lupus erythematosus. *Medicine* 60: 208–217.

Locke, S. E.; Hurst, M. W.; Heisel, J. S.; Kraus, L.; and Williams, R. M. (1979). The influence of stress and other psychosocial factors on human immunity. Presented at *American Psychosom. Soc. Meet.* (unpublished) Dept. Biol. Sci. & Psychosom. Med., Boston U. School of Medicine, Boston.

Lorber, A.; Cutler, L. S.; and Chang, C. C. (1968). Serum copper levels in rheumatoid arthritis: relationship of elevated copper to protein alterations. *Arthritis Rheum.* 11: 65–71.

Lukert, B. P., and Adams, J. S. (1976). Calcium and phosphorus homeostasis in man: effect of corticosteroids. *Arch. Intern. Med.* 136: 1249.

Lunde, G. (1970). Analysis of arsenic and selenium in marine raw materials. *J. Sci. Food Agric.* 21: 242.

Lyampert, I. M., and Davilova, T. A. (1975). Immunological phenomena associated with cross-reactive antigens of micro-organisms and mammalian tissues. *Prog. Allergy* 18: 423.

Lynch, H. T., Schuelke, G. S.; and O'Hara, M. K. (1984). Is cancer communicable? *Med. Hypotheses* 14: 181–198.

Lynch, H. T., et al. (1971). Esophageal cancer in a midwestern community. *Am. J. Gastro.* 55: 437–442.

MacCuish, A. C., and Irvine, W. J. (1975). Autoimmunological aspects of diabetes mellitus. *Clin. Endoc.* 4: 435–471.

MacLean, D., and Reichlin, S. (1981). Neuroendocrinology and the immune process, in *Psychoneuroimmunology*, Ader, R., ed., Academic Press, N.Y.

MacLennan, R. (1979). Diet and human carcinogenesis with special reference to colon cancer. *Nutrition and Cancer* 1: 42.

MacMahon, B. (1979). Dietary hypothesis concerning the etiology of human breast cancer. *Nutrition and Cancer* 1: 38.

MacMahon, B.; Cole, P.; and Brown, J. (1973). Etiology of human breast cancer: a review. *J. Natl. Cancer Inst.* 50: 21–42.

MacMahon, B., et al. (1981). Coffee and cancer of the pancreas. *N. Engl. J. Med.* 304: 630–633.

Makinodan, T., and Kay, M. M. (1980). Age influence on the immune system. *Adv. Immun.* 29: 287.

Manner, H. W., et al. (1978). Amygdalin, vitamin A and enzyme induced regression of murine mammary adenocarcinomas. *J. Manipulative Physiol. Therapeutics* 1.

Manner Metabolic Physicians (1981). Manner metabolic therapy C. *Cancer Control J.* 6: 91–94.

Martin, A. A., and Tenenbaum, F. (1980). *Diet Against Disease*. Houghton Mifflin Co., Boston.

Martin, W. (1984). Do we get too much iron? *Med. Hypotheses* 14: 131–133.

Martinez, I. (1969). Factors associated with cancer of the esophagus, mouth, and pharynx in Puerto Rico. *J. Natl. Cancer Inst.* 42: 1069–1094.

Masawe, A. E.; Muindi, T. M.; and Swai, G. B. (1974). Infections of iron deficiency and other types of anemia in the tropics. *Lancet* 2: 314–317.

Maugh, T. H. (1974). Vitamin A: potential protection from carcinogens. *Science* 186: 1198.

Mayer, K., and Pizer, H. (1983). *The AIDS Fact Book*. Bantam Books, N.Y.

McBean, L. D., and Speckmann, E. W. (1982). Diet nutrition and cancer, in *Adverse Effects of Foods*, Jelliffe, E. F. P., and Jelliffe, D. B., eds., Plenum Press, N.Y.

McCarty, M. F. (1982). Nutritional insurance supplementation and corticosteroid toxicity. *Med. Hypotheses* 9: 15–156.

McConnell, I. (1975a). Structure and function of lymphoid tissue, in *The Immune System*, Hobart, M. J., and McConnell, I., eds., Blackwell Scientific, Oxford.

———. (1975b). T and B lymphocytes, in *The Immune System*, Hobart, M. J., and McConnell, I., eds., Blackwell Scientific, Oxford.

McGrath, M. (1984). DPT vaccine: suspected cause of infant's death. *Contra Costa Times*, March 12, 1984.

McHugh, M. I., et al. (1977). Immunosuppression with polyunsaturated fatty acids in renal transplantation. *Transplantation* 24: 263–267.

McKinnon, D., and Rodgerson, E. (1973). Sorbic acid salts in vaginal candidiasis. *Obstet. Gyn.* 42: 460–465.

McLaren, D. S. (1982). Excessive nutrient intakes, in *Adverse Effects of Foods*, Jelliffe, E. F. P., and Jelliffe, D. B., eds., Plenum Press, N.Y.

McLean, A. E. M., and Magee, P. W. (1970). Increased renal carcinogenesis by dimethylnitrosamine in protein deficient rats. *Brit. J. Exptl. Pathol.* 51: 587–590.

Mertin, J., and Hunt, R. (1976). Influence of polyunsaturated fatty acids on survival of skin allografts and tumor incidence in mice. *Proc. Natl. Acad. Sci. USA* 73: 928.

Miller, J. R. A. P., and Osoba, D. (1967). Current concepts of the immunological function of the thymus. *Physiol. Rev.* 47: 437.

Miller, M. E. (1978). *Host Defenses in the Human Neonate.* Grune & Stratton, N.Y.

Mintzis, M. J., et al. (1978). Malignant melanoma in spouses. *Cancer* 42: 804.

Moertel, C.; Fleming, T.; Creagan, E.; Rubin, J.; O'Connell, M.; and Ames, M. (1985). High-dose vitamin C versus placebo in the treatment of patients with advanced cancer who have had no prior chemotherapy. *N. Engl. J. Med.* 312: 127–141.

Moneret-Vantrin, D. A. (1983). False food allergies: non-specific reactions to foodstuffs, in *Clinical Reactions to Food*, Lessof, M. H., ed., John Wiley & Sons, Chichester, England.

Moore, D. M., et al. (1970). Studies on the pathogenesis of fever. *J. Exp. Med.* 131: 179–188.

Morgan, W. P. (1981). Psychological benefits of physical activity, in *Exercise in Health and Disease,* Nagle, F. J., and Montoye, J., eds., Charles C. Thomas, Springfield, Ill.

Morgan, W. P., and Costill, D. L. (1972). Psychological characteristics of the marathon runner. *J. Sports Med. Phys. Fitness* 12: 42–46.

Morishige, F., and Murata, A. (1978). Prolongation of survival times in terminal human cancer by administration of supplemental ascorbate. *J. Int. Acad. Prev. Med.* 5: 1–8.

Morris, J. N., et al. (1973). Vigorous exercise in leisure time and the incidence of coronary heart disease. *Lancet* 1: 333–338.

Morris, V. C., and Levander, O. A. (1970). Selenium content of foods. *J. Nutr.* 100: 1383.

Moskowitz, R. (1984). Vaccine related illness. *J. Am. Inst. Homeopathy* III (4): 3–6.

Mueller, H. L. (1959). Further experiences with severe allergic reactions to insect stings. *N. Engl. J. Med.* 261: 374–377.

Murray, M. J., et al. (1982). Adverse effects of normal nutrients and foods on host resistance to disease, in *Adverse Effects of Foods,* Jelliffe, E. F. P., and Jelliffe, D. B., eds., Plenum Press, N.Y.

NAS (1972). *Human Factors in Long-Duration Spaceflight.* National Academy of Sciences, Washington, D.C.

———. (1973). *Toxicants Occurring Naturally in Foods.* National Academy of Sciences, Washington, D.C.

———. (1975). *Herbal Pharmacology in the People's Republic of China.* National Academy of Sciences, Washington, D.C.

Naitoh, P. (1976). Sleep deprivation in human subjects: a reappraisal. *Waking Sleeping* 1: 53–60.

Nauss, K. M. (1982). Vitamin A and the immune response. *Nutrition and the M.D.* 8: 1–2.

Nerup, J., and Lernmark, A. (1981). Autoimmunity in insulin-dependent diabetes mellitus. *J. Am. Med. Assoc.* 70: 135–141.

Neuhauser, I., and Gustus, E. L. (1954). Clinical use of caprylic acid. *Arch. Intern. Med.* 93: 56–60.

Neumann, C. G. (1977). Nonspecific host factors and infection in malnutrition — a review, in *Malnutrition and the Immune Response,* Suskind, R. M., ed., Raven Press, N.Y.

Newberne, P. M., and Rogers, A. E. (1973). Rat colon carcinomas associated with aflatoxin and marginal vitamin A. *J. Natl. Cancer Inst.* 50: 439–448.

Newberne, P. M., and Suphakarn, V. (1983). Nutrition and cancer: a review, with emphasis on the role of vitamins C and E and selenium. *Nutrition and Cancer* 5: 107–118.

Newberne, P. M., and Thurman, G. B. (1981). Symposium: lipids and the immune system. *Cancer Res.* 41: 3783.

Newberne, P. M., and Wilson, R. B. (1972). Prenatal malnutrition and postnatal responses in infection. *Nutr. Rept. Intern.* 5: 151–158.

New Realities (1985). Interview: Norman Cousins. *New Realities,* January/February, 8–15.

Nisonoff, A. (1971). Molecules of immunity, in *Immunobiology,* Good, R. A., and Fisher, D. W., eds., Sinauer Associates, Inc., Stamford, Conn.

Nockels, C. F. (1979). Protective effects of supplemental vitamin E against infection. *Fed. Proc.* 38: 2134–2138.

Nomura, A.; Stemmermann, G. N.; and Heilbrun, L. K. (1981). Coffee and pancreatic cancer. *Lancet* 2: 415.

Notkins, A. L. (1979). The causes of diabetes. *Sci. Am.* 241: 62–73.

O'Connor, R., et al. (1964). Death from wasp sting. *Ann. Allergy* 22: 385.

Oda, T., ed. (1976). *Hepatitis Viruses.* University Park Press, Baltimore.

Oppenheim, J. J., and Rosenstreich, D. L. (1975). Signals regulating in vitro activation of lymphocytes. *Prog. Allergy* 20: 65–94.

Paffenberger, R. S., and Hale, W. E. (1975). Work activity and coronary heart disease. *N. Engl. J. Med.* 292: 545–550.

Paffenberger, R. S.; Wing, A. L.; and Hyde, R. T. (1978). Physical activity as an index of heart attack risk in college alumni. *Am. J. Epidemiol.* 108: 161–175.

Pahwa, R., et al. (1980). Thymic function in man. *Thymus* 1: 27–58.

Palmblad, J. (1976). Fasting in man: effect on PMN granulocyte function, plasma iron and serum transferrin. *Scand. J. Haematol.* 17: 217–226.

———. (1981). Stress and immunologic competence: studies in man, in *Psychoneuroimmunology,* Ader, R., ed., Academic Press, N.Y.

Palmblad, J., et al. (1976). Stressor exposure and immunological response in man: interferon producing capacity and phagocytosis. *Psychosom. Res.* 20: 193–199.

———. (1979a). Lymphocyte and granulocyte reactions during sleep deprivation. *Psychosomatic Med* 41, 273–278.

———. (1979b). Thyroid reactions during sleep deprivation. *Acta Endocr.* 90: 233–239.

Parish, W. E. (1971). General concepts of autosensitivity in disease. *Adv. Biol. Skin.* 11: 233.

Parsons, R. M., et al. (1974). Regression of malignant tumors in magnesium and potassium depletion induced by diet and haemodialysis. *Lancet* 1: 343–344.

Passwell, J. H.; Steward, M. W.; and Soothill, J. F. (1974). The effects of protein malnutrition on macrophage function and the amount and affinity of antibody response. *Clin. Exp. Immun.* 17: 491–495.

Patterson, P. Y. (1966). Experimental allergic encephalomyelitis and autoimmune disease. *Adv. Immun.* 5: 131.

Patterson, R., ed. (1980). *Allergic Diseases.* J. B. Lippincott Co., Philadelphia.

Pelletier, K. (1979). *Holistic Medicine.* Delacorte Press, N.Y.

———. (1981). *Longevity.* Delacorte Press, N.Y.

Perper, R. J., ed. (1975). Mechanisms of tissue injury with reference to rheumatoid arthritis. *Ann. NY Acad. Sci.* 256: 5.

Peto, R.; Doll, R.; Buckley, J. D.; and Sporn, M. B. (1981). Can dietary beta-carotene materially reduce human cancer rates? *Nature* 290: 201–208.

Petrini, B., et al. (1977). Immunologic investigation in children with recurrent pneumonia. *Scand. J. Infect. Dis.* 9: 197–203.

Pihl, R. O., and Parkes, M. (1977). Hair element content in learning disabled children. *Science* 198: 204–206.

Plaut, S. M., and Friedman, S. B. (1981). Psychosocial factors in infectious disease, in *Psychoneuroimmunology*, Ader, R., ed., Academic Press, N.Y.

Podolsky, S. (1983). Diabetes and arthritis. *Diabetes Forecast,* July-August, 35-37.

Pollara, B., et al., eds. (1980). *Inborn Errors of Specific Immunity.* Academic Press, N.Y.

Pollock, M. L., et al. (1978). *Health and Fitness through Physical Activity.* John Wiley & Sons, N.Y.

Posner, B. M.; Broitman, S. A.; and Vitale, J. J. (1980). Nutrition in neoplastic disease. *Advances in Modern Human Nutrition and Dietetics* 29: 130-169.

Poston, R. N. (1979). Nutrition and immunity, in *Nutrition and Disease,* Jarrett, R. J., ed., University Park Press, Baltimore.

Prasad, J. S. (1978). *Trace Elements and Iron in Human Metabolism.* Plenum Books, N.Y.

————. (1980). Effect of vitamin E supplementation on leukocyte function. *Am. J. Clin. Nutr.* 33: 606-608.

Pritchard, M. H., and Nuki, G. (1978). Gold and penicillamine: a proposed mode of action in rheumatoid arthritis, based on synovial fluid analysis. *Annals Rheum. Dis.* 37: 493-503.

Purtilo, D. T., et al. (1976). Humoral immunity of parasitized malnourished children. *Am. J. Trop. Med.* 25: 229-232.

Raff, M. C. (1971). Surface antigenic markers for distinguishing T and B lymphocytes in mice. *Transplant Rev.* 6: 52.

Rafii, M., et al. (1977). Immune responses in malnourished children. *Clin. Immunol. Immunopathol.* 8: 1-6.

Rahe, R. H. (1972). Subject's recent life changes and near-future illness susceptibility. *Psychosom. Med.* 8: 2-19.

Raloff, J. (1983). Locks — a key to violence? *Science News* 12: 122-124.

Rasmussen, A. (1969). Emotions and immunity. *Ann. NY Acad. Sci.* 164: 45.

Rasmussen, A.; Marsh, J.; and Brill, M. (1957). Increased susceptibility to herpes simplex in mice subjected to avoidance learning stress or restraint. *Exp. Bio. Med.* 96: 183.

Rathbone, J. L. (1976). Relaxation effects of exercise, in *The Humanistic and Mental Aspects of Sports, Exercise and Recreation,* Craig, T. T., ed., American Medical Association, Chicago.

Reddy, B. S.; Narisawa, T.; and Weigburger, J. I. I. (1976). Effect of a diet with high levels of protein and fat on colon carcinogenesis in F344 rats treated with 1,2 methylhydrazine. *J. Natl. Cancer Inst.* 57: 567-569.

Reddy, V.; Raghuramulu, N.; and Bhaskaram, C. (1976). Secretory IgA in protein calorie malnutrition. *Arch. Dis. Child.* 51: 871–874.

Reinherz, E. L., and Schlossman, S. F. (1980a). The differentiation and function of human T lymphocytes. *Cell.* 19: 821–827.

———. (1980b). Regulation of the immune response — inducer and repressor T lymphocyte subsets in human beings. *N. Engl. J. Med.* 303: 370–373.

Renfrow, N. E., and Bolton, B. (1979). Personality characteristics associated with aerobic exercise in adult males. *J. Pers. Assess.* 43: 216–266.

Reuben, J. M., et al. (1983). Immunological characterization of homosexual males. *Cancer Res.* 43: 897–904.

Rimsza, M. E. (1978). Complications of corticosteroid therapy. *Am. J. Dis. Child.* 132: 806.

Rodman, T.; Laurence, J.; and Pruslin, F. (1985). Naturally occurring antibodies reactive with sperm proteins. *Science* 228: 1211–1215.

Roe, D. A. (1976). *Drug-Induced Nutritional Deficiencies.* Avi Pub. Co., Inc., Westport, Conn.

Rogers, A. E.; Herndon, B. J.; and Newberne, P. M. (1973). Induction by dimethylhydrazine of intestinal carcinoma in normal rats fed high or low levels of vitamin A. *Cancer Res.* 33: 1003–1009.

Rogers, A. E., and Newberne, P. M. (1975). Dietary effects on chemical carcinogenesis in animal models for colon and liver tumors. *Cancer Res.* 35: 3427–3431.

Rogers, A. E., et al. (1974). Enhancement of nitrosamine carcinogenesis. *Cancer Res.* 34: 96–99.

Rogers, M. P., et al. (1979). The influence of the psyche and the brain on immunity and disease susceptibility: a critical review. *Psychosom. Med.* 41: 147–165.

Rollins, Louis (1974). Moeur et coutumes des Anciens Maoris des Iles Marquises. *Stepolde* Papeete, Tahiti.

Rosch, P. J. (1979). Stress and illness. *J. Am. Med. Assoc.* 242: 427–428.

Rose, G., et al. (1974). Colon cancer and blood cholesterol. *Lancet* 1: 181–183.

Rose, N. R., and Milgrom, F. (1971). *Cellular Interactions in the Immune Response.* S. Karger, Basel.

Rose, N. R.; Milgrom, F.; and van Oss, C. J., eds. (1976). *Principles of Immunology.* Macmillan, N.Y.

Rosen, F. S. (1974). Primary immunodeficiency. *Pediatr. Clin. N. Am.* 21: 533–549.

Rosenbaum, M. (1984). Nutrients and the Immune System (unpublished manuscript).

Rossini, A. A. (1983). Self against self. *Diabetes Forecast,* July-August, 26–28.

Rowlands, L. P., ed. (1971). *Immunological Disorders of the Nervous System.* Williams & Wilkins Co., Baltimore.

Russ, J. E., and Scanlon, E. F. (1980). Identical cancer in husband and wife. *Surg. Gyn. Ob.* 150: 664.

Ryser, H. P. (1971). Chemical carcinogenesis. *N. Engl. J. Med.* 285: 721–734.

Sakane, T., et al. (1982). Effects of methyl-B$_{12}$ on the in vitro immune functions of human T lymphocytes. *J. Clin. Immunol.* 2: 101.

Samter, M., ed. (1971). *Immunological Diseases.* Little, Brown and Co., Boston.

Sandler, R. S. (1983). Diet and cancer: food additives, coffee, and alcohol. *Nutr. Cancer* 4: 273–278.

Sapse, A. T. (1984). Stress, cortisol, interferon and stress diseases. *Med. Hypotheses* 13: 31–44.

Schimke, R. N., and Kirkpatrick, C. H. (1968). Genetic studies in immunologic deficiency diseases. *Birth Defects Original Articles Series* 4: 328–339.

Schimpff, S. C., et al. (1976). Leukemia and lymphoma patients linked by prior social contact. *Ann. Int. Med.* 84: 547–550.

Schmale, A. (1958). Relationship of separation and depression to disease. *Psychosom. Med.* 204: 260.

Schwartz, R. S. (1971). Immunosuppression: the challenge of selectivity, in *Immunobiology,* Good, R. A., and Fisher, D. W., eds., Sinauer Associates, Inc., Stamford, Conn.

Scrimshaw, N. S.; Taylor, C. E.; and Gordon, J. E. (1968). Interaction of nutrition and infection. *WHO Monograph Series* 57.

Seligman, M., and Hitzig, W. H., eds. (1980). *Primary Immunodeficiencies.* Elsevier/North-Holland, Amsterdam.

Sell, S. (1980). *Immunology, Immunopathology and Immunity.* Harper & Row, Publishers, Hagerstown, Md.

Selve, H. (1956). *The Stress of Life.* McGraw-Hill Book Co., N.Y.

Shamberger, R. J., and Frost, D. V. C. (1969). Possible protective effect of selenium against human cancer. *Canadian Med. Assoc. J.* 100: 682.

Shapcott, D. (1982). Essential trace mineral deficiencies and cardiovascular disease, in *Nutrition and Killer Diseases,* Rose, J., ed., Noyes Publications, Park Ridge, N.J.

Sharma, R. P. (1981). *Immunologic Considerations in Toxicology,* Volume 1. CRC Press, Inc., Boca Raton, Fla.

Shekelle, R. B. (1981). Dietary Vitamin A and risk of cancer. *Lancet* November 28, 1981, 1185.

Schulman, S. (1971). Thyroid antigens and autoimmunity. *Adv. Immun.* 14: 85.

———. (1974). *Tissue Specificity and Autoimmunity.* Springer-Verlag, Berlin.

———. (1975). *Reproduction and Antibody Response.* CRC Press, Inc., Cleveland.

Sigel M. M., and Good, R. A., eds. (1972). *Tolerance, Autoimmunity and Aging.* Charles C. Thomas, Springfield, Ill.

Simonton, O. C.; Matthews-Simonton, S.; and Creighton, J. L. (1978). *Getting Well Again.* J. P. Tarcher, Los Angeles.

Sipes, R. G. (1976). Sports as a control for aggression, in *The Humanistic and Mental Health Aspects of Sports, Exercise and Recreation,* Craig, T. T., ed., American Medical Association, Chicago.

Smith, P. G., and Jick, H. (1978). Cancer among users of preparations containing vitamin A. *Cancer* 42: 808–811.

Smith, R. T. (1972). Possibilities and problems of immunologic intervention in cancer. *N. Engl. J. Med.* 287: 439–450.

Smolev, B. A. (1976). The relationship between sports and aggression, in *The Humanistic and Mental Health Aspects of Sports, Exercise and Recreation,* Craig, T. T., ed., American Medical Association, Chicago.

Solomon, G. F. (1981a). Emotional and personality factors in the onset and course of autoimmune disease, particularly rheumatoid arthritis, in *Psychoneuroimmunology,* Ader, R., ed., Academic Press, N.Y.

Solomon, G. F. (1981b). Immunologic abnormalities in mental illness, in *Psychoneuroimmunology,* Ader, R., ed., Academic Press, N.Y.

Solomon, G. F.; Merigan, T. C.; and Levine, S. (1967). Variations in adrenal cortical hormones within physiological ranges, stress and interferon production in mice. *Proc. Soc. Exp. Biol. Med.* 126: 74–79.

Sonnabend, J. A., and Saadoun, S. (1984). The acquired immunodeficiency syndrome: a discussion of etiologic hypotheses. *AIDS Research* 1 (2): 107–120.

Soothill, J. F. (1983). Food allergy in childhood, in *Clinical Reactions to Food,* Lessof, M. H., ed., John Wiley & Sons, Chichester, England.

Steihm, E. R. (1980). Humoral immunity in malnutrition. *Fed. Proc.* 39: 3093–3097.

Stein, M.; Schiavi, R. C.; and Camerino, M. (1976). Influence of brain and behavior on the immune system. *Science* 191: 435–440.

Stein, M.; Schleifer, S. J.; and Keller, S. E. (1981). Hypothalamic influences on immune response, in *Psychoneuroimmunology,* Ader, R., ed., Academic Press, N.Y.

Stimson, P. M., and Hodes, H. L. (1956). *A Manual of the Common Contagious Diseases.* Lea & Febinger, Philadelphia.

Strauss, A. J. (1968). Myasthenia gravis, autoimmunity and the thymus. *Adv. Intern. Med.* 14: 241.

Strom, T. B. (1982). Clinical transplantation, in *Clinical Immunology*, Stites, D. P., et al., eds., Lange, Los Altos.

Suskind, R. M., ed. (1977). *Malnutrition and the Immune Response.* Raven Press, N.Y.

Swann, P. F., and McLean, A. E. M. (1971). Cellular injury and carcinogenesis, the effect of a protein-free high-carbohydrate diet on the metabolism of dimethylnitrosamine in the rat. *Biochem. J.* 124: 283–288.

Symington, T. (1982). Nutrition and cancer, in *Nutrition and Killer Diseases*, Rose, J., ed., Noyes Publications, Park Ridge, N.J.

Sztein, M. B., et al. (1981). The role of macrophages in the acute-phase response: SAA inducer is closely related to lymphocyte activating factor and endogenous pyrogen. *Cell Immunol.* 63: 164–178.

Talal, N. (1977). *Autoimmunity: Genetic, Immunologic, Virologic, and Clinical Aspects.* Academic Press, N.Y.

Tanaka, J.; Fujiwara, H.; and Torisu, M. (1979). Enhancement of helper T cell activity by dietary supplementation of vitamin E in mice. *Immunology* 38: 727.

Tannenbaum, S. R., et al. (1978). Nitrite and nitrate are formed by endogenous synthesis in the human intestine. *Science* 220: 1487.

Tattersall, R. B., and Pike, D. A. (1972). Diabetes in identical twins. *Lancet* 2: 1120–1125.

Teas, J. (1983). Dietary intake of laminaria, a brown seaweed, and breast cancer prevention. *Nutr. Cancer* 4: 217–222.

Thal, L. J., et al. (1983). Oral physostigmine and lecithin improve memory in Alzheimer's disease. *Ann. Neurol.* 13: 491–496.

Thomas, G. S. (1981). *Exercise and Health.* Delgeschlager, Gunn and Hain, Publishers, Inc., Cambridge, England.

Thomas, W. R., and Holt, P. G. (1978). Vitamin C and immunity: an assessment of the evidence. *Clin. Exp. Immunol.* 32: 370–379.

Truesdell, D.; Whitney, E.; and Acosta, P. (1984). Nutrients in vegetarian foods. *J. Amer. Diet. Assoc.* 84 (1): 28–35.

Tulinius, H. (1979). Epidemiology of gastric cancer. *Nutr. Cancer* 1: 61.

Turnbridge, W. M. G., et al. (1977). The spectrum of thyroid diseases in a community: the Wickham survey. *Clin. Endoc.* 7: 481.

Turner, R. W. D. (1982). Diet and epidemic coronary heart disease, in *Nutrition and Killer Diseases*, Rose, J., ed., Noyes Publications, Park Ridge, N.J.

Turpeinen, O. (1979). Effect of cholesterol-lowering diet on mortality from coronary heart disease and other causes. *Circulation* 59: 1–7.

Tuyns, A. J.; Pequijnot, G.; and Abbatuici, J. S. (1979). Esophageal cancer and alcohol consumption: importance of type of beverage. *Brit. J. Cancer* 23: 443–447.

Ugai, K.; Ziff, M.; and Lipsky, P. E. (1979). Gold-induced changes in the morphology and functional capabilities of human monocytes. *Arthritis Rheum.* 22: 1352–1360.

Ulett, G. A. (1980). Food allergy — cytotoxic testing and the central nervous system. *Psychiatric J. Univ. Ottawa* 5: 100–108.

USDA: Watt, B. K., and Merrill, A. L. (1963). *Composition of foods. Agric. Hdbk. No. 8.,* U.S. Dept. of Agriculture.

Utsumi, H., and Elkind, M. M. (1983). Caffeine-enhanced survival of radiation-sensitive repair-deficient Chinese hamster cells. *Rad. Res.* 96: 348–358.

Vischer, T. L. (1971). Immunologic aspects of chronic hepatitis. *Prog. Allergy* 15: 268.

Vistainer, M., et al. (1982). *Science* 216: 437–440.

Vitale, J. J. (1975). Possible role of nutrients in neoplasia. *Cancer Res.* 35: 3320–3325.

Vitale, J. J., and Good, R. A., eds. (1974). Nutrition and immunology. Symposium on nutrition and immunology. *Am. J. Clin. Nutr.* 27: 623–669.

Vyas, G. M.; Stites, D. P.; and Brecher, G., eds. (1975). *Laboratory Diagnosis of Immunological Disorders.* Grune & Stratton, N.Y.

Wald, N.; Idle, M.; and Boreham, J. (1980). Low serum vitamin A and subsequent risk of cancer. *Lancet,* October 18, 1980, 813.

Walford, R. L. (1969). *The Immunologic Theory of Aging.* Einar Munksgaard, Copenhagen.

Weinberg, E. O. (1971). Roles of iron on host-parasite interactions. *J. Infect. Diseases* 124: 401–409.

———. (1983). Iron in neoplastic disease. *Nutrition and Cancer* 4: 223–232.

Weiner, M. A. (1980). *Weiner's Herbal.* Stein & Day, N.Y.

———. (1981). *The Way of the Skeptical Nutritionist.* Macmillan, N.Y.

———. (1983). *Getting Off Cocaine.* Avon Books, N.Y.

Weiner, M. A., and Goss, K. (1982). *The Complete Book of Homeopathy.* Bantam, N.Y.

———. (1983). *Nutrition against Aging.* Bantam, N.Y.

Weisburd, S. (1984). Food for mind and mood. *Science News* 125: 216–219.

Weksler, M. E. (1981). The senescence of the immune system. *Hospital Practice* 16: 53.

Whittingham, S. (1972). Serological methods in autoimmune disease in man. *Res. Immunochem. Immunobiol.* 1: 123.

Williams, R. J. (1975). *Physician's Handbook of Nutritional Science.* Charles C. Thomas, Springfield, Ill.

Williams, R. R., and Horm, J. W. (1977). Association of cancer sites with tobacco and alcohol consumption and socioeconomic status of patients: interview study from the third national cancer survey. *J. Natl. Cancer Inst.* 58: 525–547.

Williams, R. R., et al. (1981). Cancer incidence by levels of cholesterol. *J. Am. Med. Assoc.* 245: 247–252.

Winick, M. (1969). Malnutrition and brain development. *J. Pediatr.* 74: 667–679.

Witkin, S.; Bongiovanni, A.; and Yu, I. (1983). Humoral immune responses in healthy heterosexual, homosexual and vasectomized men and in homosexual men with AIDS. *AIDS Research* 1 (1): 31–44.

Wittig, H. J., et al. (1970). *A Primer on Immunologic Disorders.* Charles C. Thomas, Springfield, Ill.

Wolf, G. (1982). Is dietary B-carotene an anti-cancer agent? *Nutrition Review 40: 257–261.*

Worthington, B. S. (1974). Effect of nutritional status on immune phenomena. J. Amer. Diet. Assoc. 65: 123.

Wyburn-Mason, R. (1978). *The Causation of Rheumatoid Disease and Many Human Cancers.* IJI Publ. Co., Ltd., Tokyo.

Wynder, E. L. (1975). The epidemiology of large bowel cancer. *Cancer Res.* 35: 3388–3394.

Wynder, E. L.; Escher, G.; and Mantel, N. (1966). An epidemiologic investigation of cancer of the endometrium. *Cancer* 19: 489–520.

Wynder, E. L., et al. (1969). Environmental factors of cancer of the colon and rectum. II. Japanese epidemiological data. *Cancer* 23: 1210–1220.

———. (1973). Epidemiology of cancer of the pancreas. *J. Natl. Cancer Inst.* 50: 645–667.

Yoon, J. W., et al. (1979). Virus-induced diabetes mellitus: isolation of a virus from the pancreas of a child with diabetic ketoacidosis. *N. Engl. J. Med.* 300: 1173–1179.

Yunis, E. J., and Greenberg, L. J. (1974). Immunopathology of aging. *Fed. Proc.* 33: 2017–2019.

Zajicek, G. (1984). On the declining cancer rate. *Med. Hypotheses* 13: 123–124.

Ziff, M., ed. (1973). Models for the study and therapy of rheumatoid arthritis. *Fed. Proc.* 32: 131.

Zvaifler, N. J. (1973). The immunopathology of joint inflammation in rheumatoid arthritis. *Adv. Immun.* 16: 265.

Index

Acetylcholine, 67, 69, 70; choline in stimulating, 70
Acidosis, 220
Active Meditation, 206
Ader, R., 52, 126, 286
Adrenalin, 46, 67
Ahlqvist, J., 64, 286
AIDS (Acquired Immune Deficiency Syndrome), 159, 165, 181, 184–85, 229; causes for, 190–93; and chronic thrush, 233; communicability, 207–10; controlling, 210–12; defined, 184–85; diseases associated with, 194–95, 233; epidemiology for, 188; in Europe, 188–91; heterosexual, 208–9; politics with, 212–13; prevention, 197–98; reducing risk of contracting, 184–213; in remission, 201–7; reported cases, 181, 187; risk groups, 186, 191; secondary infections with, 209–10, 233; and stress management, 59; symptoms, 193; T helpers to T suppressors ratio in, 24; transmission, 187, 207–9; vitamin C for, 150; *see also* HTLV-III virus; Kaposi's sarcoma
Akhtar, H., 19, 286
Alcohol, 82–83
Alkylating agents, 230
Allergens: in allergy testing, 251; defined, 284; food, 85–88; IgE complex, 244–45; removing, 252
Allergies: asthma, 245–46; clinical ecology treatment for, 252–53; drug, 249–50; ear, 246; eye, 246; food, 85–88, 248–49; hay fever, 244–45; immunity against, 243–53; to insects, 246–47; nutrition for treating, 252; rhinitis, 244–45; testing for, 251
Alzheimer's disease, 67, 70; acetylcholine in treating, 70
Amebiasis, 156
American Academy of Pediatrics, 161
American Cancer Society, 15, 66
Amino acids, 33, 263–64; in antibodies, 33; in boosting neurotransmitters, 68–71; choline, 69; as dietary supplements, 70–71; "essential," 264; lack-

(Amino acids, *cont.*)
ing in, and malnutrition, 88–90; phenylalanine, 74–75; tryptophan, 69, 70; tyrosine, 69, 70; vitamins for utilizing, 70
Amoebas, 217
Anaphylactic reaction, 246–48; to drugs, 250; to insect bites, 246–47
Anaphylactic shock, 247
Antibiotics, 149–50
Antibodies (IG's), 22, 26, 33–34, 145, 284; acquiring, 36–37; AIDS, 188; antibrain, 63; and antigens, 56–57; antinuclear, 221; in aspermatogenesis, 222; combining sites in, 33; from B cells, 145; to hinder bacterial toxins, 151; defined, 284; effect of malnutrition on, 89; five types of, 33–34; function of (Tables), 31, 34; germline theory for, 36; HTLV-III, 211; humoral, 166–67; IgE, 244; and immunization, 159; location of (Table), 31; in myasthenia gravis, 222; production, 23–24; in rheumatoid arthritis, 216; riboflavin in producing, 101; in schizophrenics, 63; in scleroderma, 221; somatic mutation theory for, 36; sperm, 196; in systemic lupus erythematosus, 218; from T cells, 145; in transplant rejection, 166; *see also* Antigens; B cells; Immunoglobulin; Lymphocytes; T cells
Antibrain antibodies, 63
Antigenic drift, 145
Antigens, 18–19, 26, 33, 151; in anaphylaxis, 247; in autoimmune diseases, 223–24; Ia (immune-associated), 220; AIDS, 210–11; and antibodies, 33–34, 56–57; histocompatibility, 167; and immune memory, 33–34; in interferon production, 171; and lymph nodes, 29; and sperm immunosuppression, 196; tumor, 171; in vaccine, 35, 159; *see also* Antibodies; Macrophages
Anti-immunity foods, 87

· 317 ·